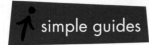
simple guides

Arthritis

Dr Eleanor Bull
Dr Paul Creamer

Arthritis
First published – April 2006

Published by
CSF Medical Communications Ltd
1 Bankside, Lodge Road, Long Hanborough
Oxfordshire, OX29 8LJ, UK
T +44 (0)1993 885370 F +44 (0)1993 881868
enquiries@bestmedicine.com
www.bestmedicine.com

We are always interested in hearing from anyone
who has anything to add to our Simple Guides.
Please send your comments to *editor@csfmedical.com*.

Author Dr Eleanor Bull
Managing Editor Dr Eleanor Bull
Medical Editor Dr Paul Creamer
Science Editor Dr Scott Chambers
Production Editor Emma Catherall
Layout Jamie McCansh and Julie Smith
Operations Manager Julia Savory
Publisher Stephen I'Anson

ISBN-10: 1-905466-12-9
ISBN-13: 978-190546-612-2

Printed in Italy.

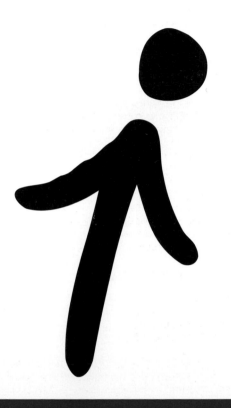

FOREWORD

TRISHA MACNAIR
Doctor and BBC Health Journalist

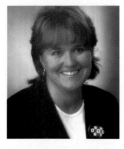 Getting involved in managing your own medical condition – or helping those you love or care for to manage theirs – is a vital step towards keeping as healthy as possible.

Whilst doctors, nurses and the rest of your healthcare team can help you with expert advice and guidance, nobody knows your body, your symptoms and what is right for *you* as well as you do.

There is no long-term (chronic) medical condition or illness that I can think of where the person concerned has absolutely no influence at all on their situation. The way you choose to live your life, from the food you eat to the exercise you take, will impact upon your disease, your well-being and how able you are to cope. You are in charge!

Being involved in making choices about your treatment helps you to feel in control of your problems, and makes sure you get the help that you really need. Research clearly shows that when people living with a chronic illness take an active role in looking after themselves, they can bring about significant improvements in their illness and vastly improve the quality of life they enjoy.

Of course, there may be occasions when you feel particularly unwell and it all seems out of your control. Yet most of the time there are plenty of things that you can do in order to reduce the negative effects that your condition can have on your life. This way you feel as good as possible and may even be able to alter the course of your condition.

So how do you gain the confidence and skills to take an active part in managing your condition, communicate with health professionals and work through sometimes worrying and emotive issues? The answer is to become better informed. Reading about your problem, talking to others who have been through similar experiences and hearing what the experts have to say will all help to build up your understanding and help you to take an active role in your own health care.

Simple Guides provide an invaluable source of help, giving you the facts that you need in order to understand the key issues and discuss them with your doctors and other professionals involved in your care. The information is presented in an accessible way but without neglecting the important details. Produced independently and under the guidance of medical experts *Arthritis* is an evidence-based, balanced and up-to-date review that I hope you will find enables you to play an active part in the successful management of your condition.

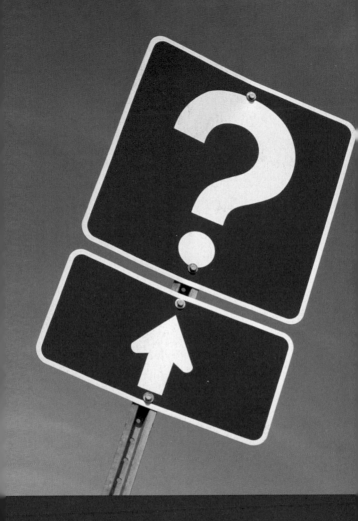

What happens normally?

WHAT HAPPENS NORMALLY?

Our joints hold our skeleton together and give us flexibility. Without them, we would be unable to move at all.

WHAT IS A JOINT?

Put simply, a joint is the point at which two bones meet. There are three major types of joint.

1. Immovable (or fibrous). As their name suggests, these joints don't move! The plates of bone that make up our skull are linked together by this type of joint.

2. Partially moveable (or cartilaginous; pronounced *kar-tuh-lah-juh-nus*). These joints move a little, but not very much. A good example is the sacroiliac joint in the pelvis – this joint only moves a few millimetres but is important in allowing the pelvis to 'spring' when we walk or run. The vertebrae that make up our spine are linked by cartilaginous joints.

3. Freely movable (or synovial; pronounced *sih-no-vee-ul*). These joints can move in many different directions. Most of the joints in the body are synovial joints, and they come in many shapes and sizes. The hip, shoulders, elbows, knees, wrists and ankles are all synovial joints. It is this type of joint that we will concentrate on in this book.

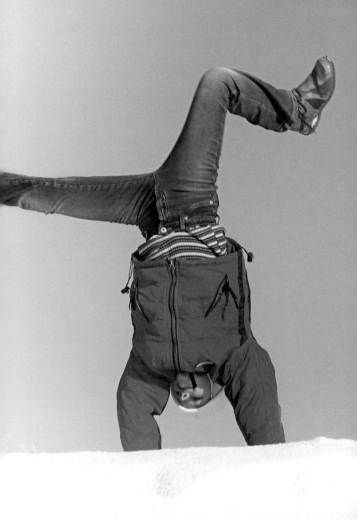

SYNOVIAL JOINTS

There are many different types of synovial joint, listed below are a few.

- Hinge joints (e.g. elbow and knee) open and close like hinges and allow movement in one direction only.

- Ball and socket joints (e.g. hip and shoulder) allow rotating and swinging movements. The round end of a long bone (e.g. the thigh bone, or femur) fits neatly into the hollow of another bone (e.g. the hipbone, or pelvis).

- Pivot joints (e.g. the neck) allow twisting movement, such as moving your head from side-to-side.

- Ellipsoid joints (e.g. at base of finger) are similar to ball and socket joints but do not have quite as much swinging and rotation.

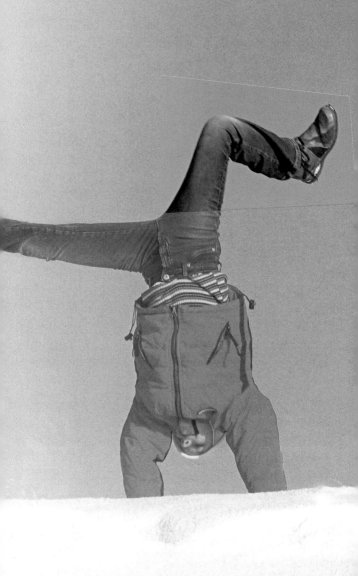

MOST OF THE JOINTS IN THE BODY ARE SYNOVIAL JOINTS.

'Synovial' comes from the Latin word for 'egg' and relates to the egg-like consistency of the thick, stringy fluid that fills and cushions the joint as it moves – the synovial fluid. Look at the structure of the synovial joint in the diagram. Synovial joints share certain features, like cartilage, the joint capsule, the synovium, ligaments and tendons.

■ **Muscle**
   The muscle powers the movement of the joint.

■ **Bone**
   Our bones are our body's scaffolding. Bones help to protect and anchor our internal organs, as well as storing calcium and other minerals, and producing blood cells.

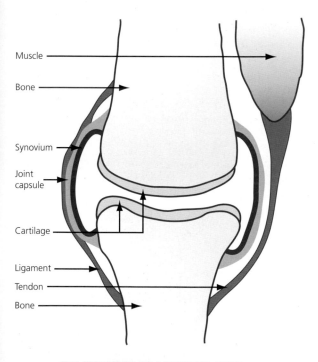

Muscle

Bone

Synovium

Joint capsule

Cartilage

Ligament

Tendon

Bone

THE STRUCTURE OF A SYNOVIAL JOINT.

■ **Synovium**
The inner layer of the joint capsule. Consists of a slippery surface that lubricates the joint and helps it to move more easily. The synovium produces the synovial fluid that fills the joint capsule, which lubricates the joint and helps to keep the cartilage slippery.

■ **Joint capsule**
The 'bag' in which the whole joint is contained. Has a tough outer layer that helps to contain the joint and stops it from losing its shape.

■ **Cartilage**
A thin layer of tough material that covers the end of the two bones forming the joint. Cartilage acts as a 'shock absorber' to cushion the joint and also helps the joint to move smoothly.

■ **Ligaments**
Thick strong bands that hold the joint together.

■ **Tendons**
Strong cords that attach the muscles to the bones on either side of the joint and help to keep the joint in place.

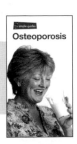

For more information see
Osteoporosis

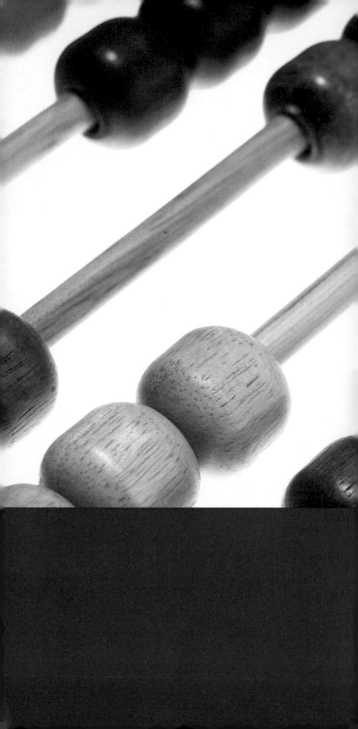

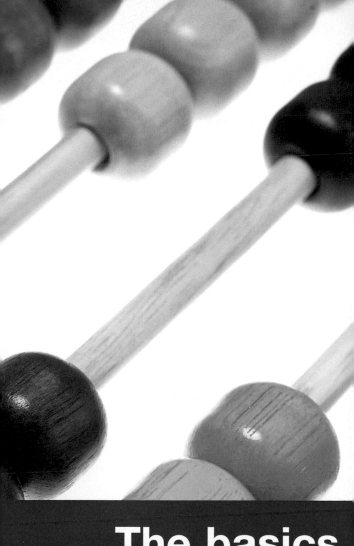

The basics

ARTHRITIS – THE BASICS

Arthritis is the name given to diseases that bring about pain in our joints. Diseases that affect our joints also govern how mobile we are and therefore how independent we are. Managing arthritis effectively is all about controlling pain and stiffness and staying as active as possible.

WHAT IS ARTHRITIS AND WHY IS IT A PROBLEM?

Arthritis is a collection of distinct diseases that all cause pain in the joints. It is usually accompanied by swelling and sometimes changes in the structure of the joint. There are as many as 100 different types of arthritis. Some of these may affect not only the joints but other parts of the body (like the skin) as well.

People who have arthritis often have trouble moving and experience some loss of function (for example, trouble with fastening clothing or performing simple household chores or other everyday tasks). This has a number of knock-on effects, to the extent that (if it is not managed properly) arthritis can end up compromising your:

- mobility
- independence
- self-confidence
- sense of well-being
- family life.

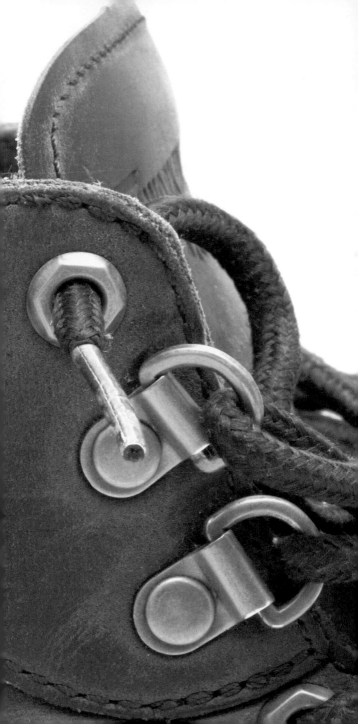

OSTEOARTHRITIS AND RHEUMATOID ARTHRITIS

Osteoarthritis and rheumatoid arthritis are the two most common types of arthritis (and are the main focus of this Simple Guide).

■ **Osteoarthritis**
Occurs when the cushioning of the joint (from the cartilage and synovial fluid) starts to wear down and disappear. The two bones of the joint start to rub together when the joint moves, which can be very painful.

■ **Rheumatoid arthritis**
Occurs when the joint as a whole becomes inflamed and swollen as a result of underlying autoimmune disease.

People with rheumatoid arthritis can often end up developing osteoarthritis eventually, because once a joint has been damaged (e.g. by rheumatoid arthritis) it becomes more susceptible to developing what is known as 'secondary osteoarthritis'.

Rheumatoid arthritis is an autoimmune disease

Our immune system protects us from foreign invaders (such as bacteria and viruses) by destroying them with specially tailored substances called antibodies.

Under normal circumstances our immune system helps to protect us against infection and without it we would not survive. However, if you have an autoimmune disease, your body mistakes healthy cells, organs, or tissues in the body for foreign invaders and starts attacking them.

If you have rheumatoid arthritis, your immune system mistakes one or more of your joints for a foreign invader and attacks it. This causes inflammation, and it is the inflammation that damages the joint and brings about the symptoms of arthritis.

Many other diseases are also autoimmune, such as some types of diabetes, anaemia, and some thyroid conditions.

For more information see
Thyroid disorders

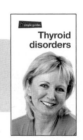

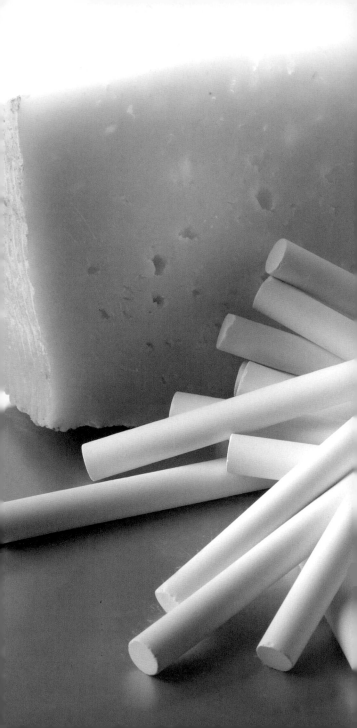

WHAT'S THE DIFFERENCE BETWEEN OSTEOARTHRITIS AND RHEUMATOID ARTHRITIS?

Although they share a name and have many symptoms in common, osteoarthritis and rheumatoid arthritis are in fact very different diseases.

- **They are caused by different things.** Although both conditions involve the breakdown of cartilage in the joint, osteoarthritis is largely due to age-related changes in which the cartilage becomes thinner in some joints, whereas rheumatoid arthritis is related to a problem with the body's own immune system.

- **They affect people of different ages.** Osteoarthritis tends to affect people as they get older and rarely occurs before the age of 40, but rheumatoid arthritis can occur at any age (and usually tends to affect people between the ages of 30 and 50 but can sometimes even start during childhood).

■ **They can affect different joints.**
Osteoarthritis mostly affects the weight-bearing joints (like the knees and the hips) whilst rheumatoid arthritis tends to affect the smaller joints (such as those in the hands, wrist or elbows). Rheumatoid arthritis is a symmetrical disease. This means that if one wrist is affected then it is likely that the other one will be too, but this is not always the case in osteoarthritis.

■ **They develop at different rates.**
Whilst osteoarthritis can take many years to develop, rheumatoid arthritis can come on over a period of months.

■ **They look different in X-rays.**
Bones affected by osteoarthritis can show bony lumps and other deformities, whereas bones affected by rheumatoid arthritis can look thin and the joints may show signs of damage ('erosions') due to the inflammation.

WHAT'S THE DIFFERENCE BETWEEN OSTEOARTHRITIS AND OSTEOPOROSIS?

Both conditions are more common in elderly than in younger people, but where osteoarthritis affects the joints, osteoporosis is specifically a problem with the strength of the bones. As the bones become progressively weaker, they are more prone to fracture. This means that a minor fall, for example, which would not normally cause a healthy bone to break, can cause a painful and debilitating fracture.

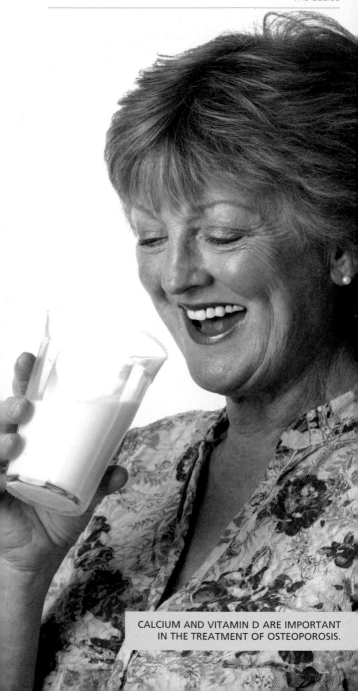

CALCIUM AND VITAMIN D ARE IMPORTANT
IN THE TREATMENT OF OSTEOPOROSIS.

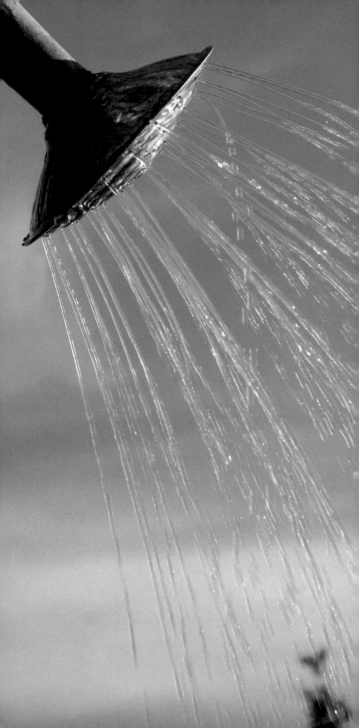

THE SYMPTOMS OF OSTEOARTHRITIS

The major symptoms of osteoarthritis are:

- pain (that gets worse after exercising or towards the end of the day)

- stiffness (that is usually worse in the mornings and after long periods of sitting down).

The symptoms of osteoarthritis usually come on gradually and you may only end up noticing them at certain times of the day (e.g. in the morning when you first get up) or after doing certain activities (e.g. weight-bearing exercises like walking or jogging). You may start to notice that your joints aren't as flexible as they used to be and that your range of movement is impaired (i.e. you can't straighten your leg out in front of you as far as you used to be able to). Performing certain activities like bending down, kneeling, gardening or climbing stairs may also start to become more difficult.

As osteoarthritis becomes more advanced, you may start to notice other symptoms like:

- muscle weakness

- swelling around the joints

- a crunching feeling in the joints

- pain during the night that keeps you awake

- changes in the outward appearance of the joint, for example they may start to look knobbly.

THE SYMPTOMS OF RHEUMATOID ARTHRITIS

Rheumatoid arthritis tends to follow a different course in different people and symptoms can even vary from one day to the next. Given the right treatment, the symptoms of rheumatoid arthritis can disappear altogether, but this is not always the case and some people's symptoms will continue to get steadily worse, even when they are receiving treatment.

Rheumatoid arthritis can affect any synovial joint (but tends to affect the smaller joints like the wrists, elbows and fingers) and interestingly

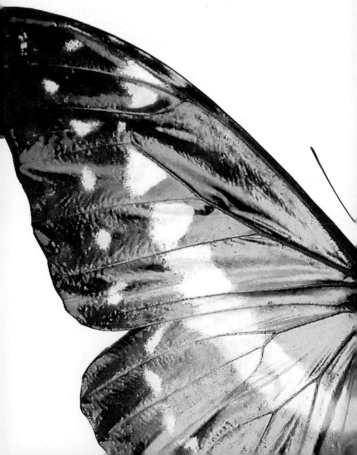

enough, is usually symmetrical (if one wrist is affected, it is more than likely that the other one will be too).

In contrast to osteoarthritis, the symptoms of rheumatoid arthritis can affect the whole body rather than just the joint in question. The main symptoms of rheumatoid arthritis are:

- pain
- stiffness
- swelling around the joints
- warmness and redness around the joints
- lumps under the skin (called rheumatoid nodules)
- tiredness
- loss of appetite.

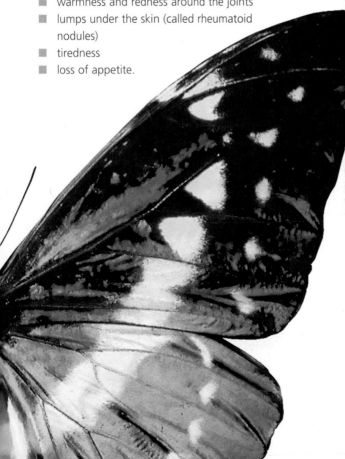

DIAGNOSING ARTHRITIS

Depending on the type of arthritis, your symptoms can develop over a matter of weeks or it may take many months before they start to bother you to the extent that you go and see your doctor for advice. If you suspect that you may have a form of arthritis, it is important that you seek medical advice as soon as you can. There is no specific test that doctors can use to diagnose arthritis. Usually, your doctor will be able to work out what's wrong by:

- listening to you describe your symptoms
- examining your joints
- examining your range of movement
- looking at your medical history
- looking at the medical history of your family
- requesting certain tests (e.g. blood tests, X-rays or scans).

Sometimes, your doctor may refer you to a specialist (called an orthopaedic surgeon or a rheumatologist) for further tests. If you are diagnosed with rheumatoid arthritis, your condition will usually be managed by a rheumatologist in a specialist clinic rather than by your GP.

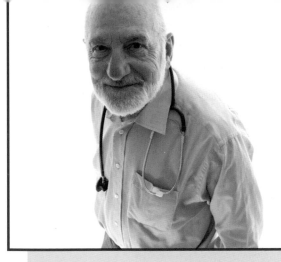

GP

As your GP, I will be responsible for co-ordinating your care in the long-term. You may come and see me because you are concerned that you may have arthritis, in which case I may sometimes refer you for further diagnostic tests at the hospital.

Alternatively, you may have already been diagnosed with arthritis and want advice about an aspect of your recommended programme of care. As well as prescribing you medications, I can offer you advice, reassurance and further explanation should you require it. I may refer you to a hospital-based specialist at any point, especially if your arthritis is proving particularly difficult to control or is very advanced. I will work with other members of the healthcare team to ensure that regular reviews and check-ups are arranged for you. I can also put you in touch with other healthcare professionals like physiotherapists and occupational therapists.

My overall aim is to tailor the management process to suit your individual circumstances. Developing and maintaining long-term relationships with my patients and their families allows me to do this.

MANAGING ARTHRITIS

Once you have been diagnosed with arthritis, your doctor will recommend an appropriate course of treatment. Bear in mind that there is usually no cure for arthritis. Current treatments can help to relieve pain and can sometimes be used to slow down the course of the disease, but if your pain persists, you will probably need to take some form of medication on and off for the rest of your life.

For rheumatoid arthritis in particular, it is important that you start treatment as early as possible. The earlier it is started, the faster it can get to work. This means that less damage can occur to the joint and will make it easier for you to get around (for longer).

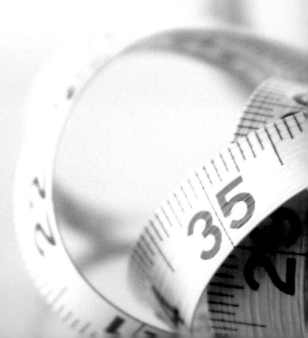

The aims of any arthritis treatment programme are:

■ to reduce pain, stiffness and swelling in the joints

■ to reduce damage to joints

■ to help people stay doing the things they want to for as long as possible.

It may involve:

■ taking regular exercise

■ losing weight (if you are overweight)

■ taking medication

■ trying a complementary or alternative therapy

■ undergoing joint replacement surgery (for a small number of people)

■ a mixture of any of the above.

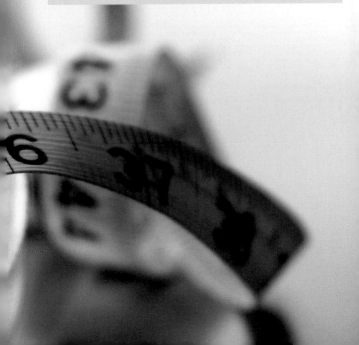

THINGS YOU CAN DO YOURSELF

Pain and stiffness can take their toll on your sense of independence. As your arthritis gradually worsens, you may find it more difficult to get around or to perform relatively simple tasks like getting dressed or doing the housework.

We will look at this in more detail later on in the book (see *Why me?* page 40) but introducing some of the following measures may help:

- fitting grab rails up stairways, in the bath or next to the toilet

- fitting higher work surfaces and raising electrical sockets up the wall so that you don't need to bend so much

- using tap-turners and contour grips to help with turning dials or knobs

- using lightweight kitchen equipment and wide-handled kitchen utensils

- shopping for your groceries on the internet and having them delivered to your door.

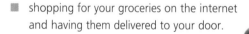

PAIN RELIEF FOR ARTHRITIS

If your arthritis is causing you pain, your doctor
may suggest some pain management strategies.
These may include:

- 'analgesic' (pain-killing) drugs, given by
  mouth, injection or in patch form

- physiotherapy, including exercises in water
  (hydrotherapy)

- transcutaneous electrical nerve stimulation
  (TENS), which interrupts the pain signals
  travelling to your brain by means of electrode
  pads attached to the skin

- complementary therapies (including
  acupuncture and massage).

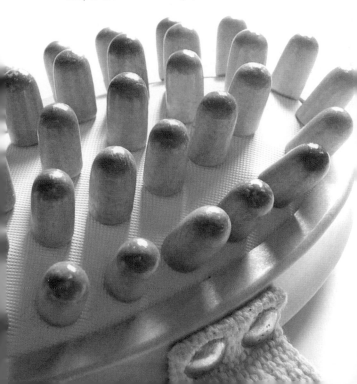

DISEASE-MODIFYING DRUGS FOR RHEUMATOID ARTHRITIS

These drugs, called disease-modifying antirheumatic drugs (DMARDs), can help to slow down the progress of rheumatoid arthritis by reducing inflammation and by reducing the activity of the body's immune system. They can reduce the rate at which joints become damaged and thereby help you to stay mobile for longer. You can take painkillers as well as DMARDs – they work well together. You will usually only be given DMARDs by a rheumatologist.

There are many different types of DMARDs, but in the UK, sulphasalazine (Salazopyrin®) and methotrexate (Matrex®) are the ones used most frequently. Other types include gold (e.g. Myocrisin®, Ridaura®), D-penicillamine, azathioprine (Imuran®), cyclophosphamide, ciclosporin-A and leflunomide (Arava®).

The 'biologic' drugs are a relatively new group of drugs to be used in the treatment of rheumatoid arthritis. They include etanercept (Enbrel®), infliximab (Remicade®) and adalimumab (Humira®) and can be given in combination with some of the DMARDs mentioned previously.

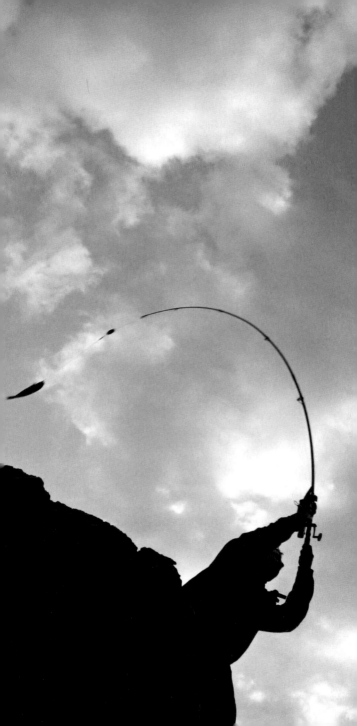

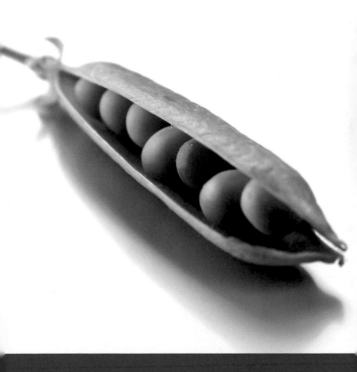

Why me?

WHY ME?

If you have arthritis, or are caring for someone with the condition, you are certainly not alone. Arthritis is the single biggest cause of physical disability in the UK.

HOW COMMON IS ARTHRITIS?

The answer is 'very common indeed'. It has been estimated that arthritis is the reason for one-in-five visits to the doctor and that 9 million people seek medical advice for arthritis each year. That's 15% of the UK population. Of the two major types of arthritis (osteo- and rheumatoid arthritis), osteoarthritis is by far the most common.

- Osteoarthritis is more common in people over the age of 60 and as the population of the UK gets older, the number of people who suffer from osteoarthritis will also increase.

- In contrast, rheumatoid arthritis can affect people of any age, and is usually first picked up between your 30s and 50s. About one in every hundred people is affected by rheumatoid arthritis, with women up to three-times more likely to suffer than men.

Osteoarthritis is much more common than rheumatoid arthritis and tends to affect older people.

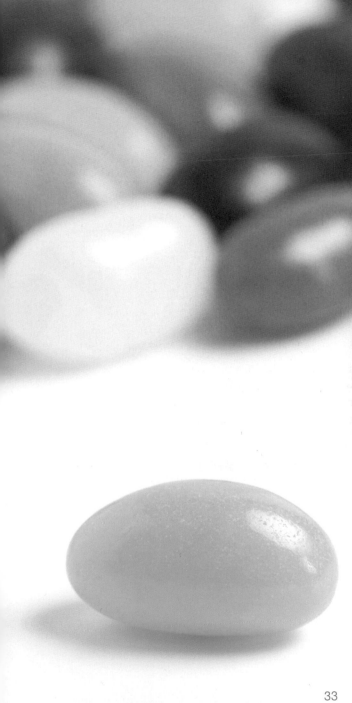

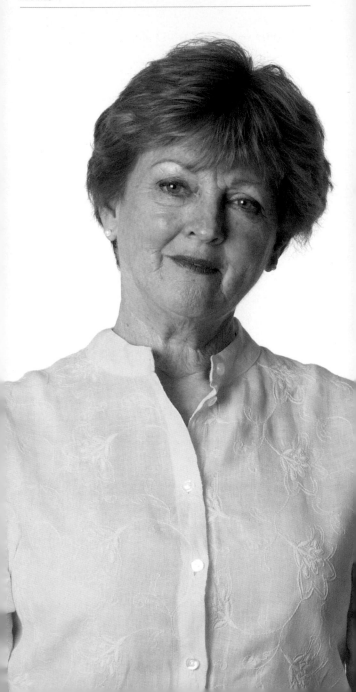

HOW DID I END UP WITH OSTEOARTHRITIS?

In the past, osteoarthritis was wrongly considered to be an unavoidable consequence of wear and tear on the joints. We now know that joints don't just wear out with age, so if you do develop osteoarthritis, it can usually be traced back to at least one (and possibly a few) of the causes listed below.

- **Growing older**
  The chances of getting osteoarthritis seem to increase with age.

- **Being overweight**
  Carrying extra weight can put joints (especially the knees and hips) under unnecessary stress and can damage them, leading to osteoarthritis.

- **Injury**
  Sustaining an injury to a joint (like a fracture) can make you more likely to develop osteoarthritis in the future. Some professional athletes can injure the same joints over and over again.

- **Your occupation**
  Performing certain tasks on a regular basis can put your joints under strain. Farmers often develop osteoarthritis in their hips and people who operate machinery like pneumatic drills can develop arthritis in their hands or elbows.

■ **Damage from another joint disease**
Suffering from a joint-damaging disease like
rheumatoid arthritis can make you more likely
to develop osteoarthritis in later years.

■ **Your family history**
Some forms of osteoarthritis do run in
families, especially those cases that affect the
small joints of fingers. But in general, heredity
is not a major reason for developing
osteoarthritis.

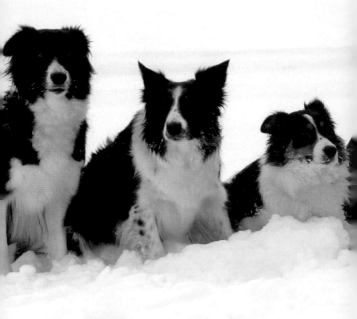

■ **Your gender**
In most joints, especially the knees and hands,
osteoarthritis is more common and severe
in women.

■ **Your anatomy**
Being born with abnormal anatomy (like
having one leg slightly longer than the other)
can make you more susceptible to developing
osteoarthritis. This is called a congenital
abnormality, because you are born with it.

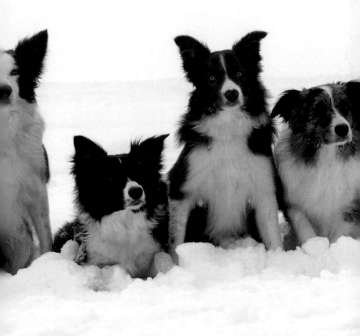

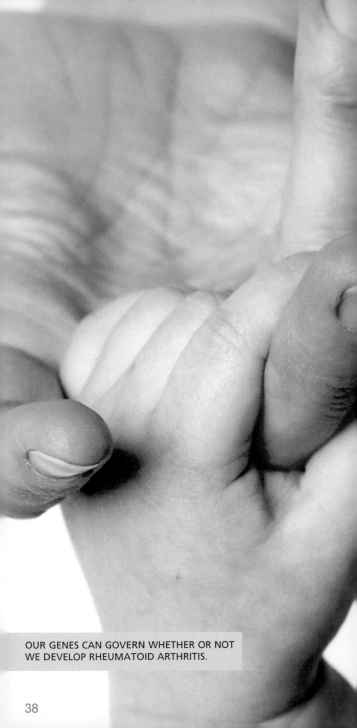

OUR GENES CAN GOVERN WHETHER OR NOT
WE DEVELOP RHEUMATOID ARTHRITIS.

HOW DID I END UP WITH RHEUMATOID ARTHRITIS?

Unlike osteoarthritis, if you develop rheumatoid arthritis in all probability there would have been very little you could have done to prevent it. In many cases the actual cause of rheumatoid arthritis is unknown. Scientists simply do not know enough about the condition to point the finger at any one particular factor, but some of those listed below may contribute.

- **Genetic factors**
  We have seen that rheumatoid arthritis is an autoimmune disease that occurs when the body's own immune system starts attacking the tissues of the body's own joints. Our genetic make-up is determined before we are born, and with it, our susceptibility to developing rheumatoid arthritis.

- **Infection**
  Some scientists believe that it is possible that being exposed to or infected with a particular bacteria or a virus could trigger the autoimmune response and ultimately lead to rheumatoid arthritis (although nobody has been able to show exactly what this infecting agent is).

- **Hormones**
  Rheumatoid arthritis is more common in women than in men, and this may be linked to different levels of different hormones. Furthermore, the disease can go into remission during pregnancy, only to relapse afterwards. There is also some evidence that those women who take the contraceptive pill are at less risk of developing rheumatoid arthritis.

ARTHRITIS AND THE HOME

Relatively simple things like getting around the house, writing letters, opening jars or doing up buttons can all become more difficult if you have arthritis. Listed below are a number of changes that you can make to your home that may help to make life a bit easier.

- Fit grab rails up stairways, in the bath or next to the toilet.

- Remove loose mats and make sure your house is well lit. This can reduce your chances of having a fall.

- Fit higher work surfaces and raise electrical sockets up the wall so that you don't need to bend so much.

- Hands-free or voice-activated telephones can help to make life easier.

- Electrically operated reclining chairs, bath or stair lifts can make it easier to get around.

- Tap-turners and contour grips can help with turning dials or knobs.
- Use lightweight kitchen equipment and wide-handled kitchen utensils.
- Buy previously chopped vegetables to avoid having to use sharp knives.
- Shop for your groceries on the internet and have them delivered to your door.

This list is by no means exhaustive. Contact your GP or your local council for details of the numerous gadgets and services (like shopmobility schemes) that are available in your area (there is also a list of contact information at the back of this book; see *Simple extras* page 128).

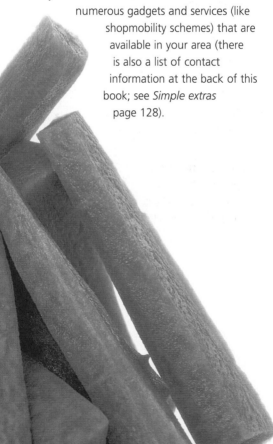

ARTHRITIS AND THE WORKPLACE

Because arthritis is so common, it stands to reason that many people of working age will be affected by it.

Although having a long-term condition like arthritis need not adversely affect your working life, many people find that it does. One sobering statistic suggests that 40% of people with rheumatoid arthritis leave work within 5 years of being diagnosed. If you do find that your arthritis is starting to affect your work, the worst thing you can do is to keep it to yourself.

Talk to other people about the problems you are experiencing, be they your colleagues, your boss, an occupational health advisor (if you have one) or even a disability employment advisor (contactable through your local Jobcentre Plus; *www.jobcentreplus.gov.uk*).

There are many things that can be done to help you overcome the difficulties you are experiencing.

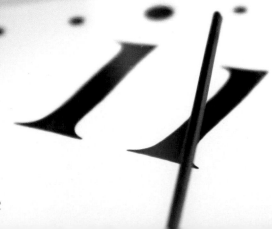

MEASURES THAT CAN HELP YOU TO DEAL WITH ARTHRITIS AT WORK

- Ask to work from home (if possible) during those periods when your symptoms are flaring up.
- Shorter or adjusted working hours (e.g. if your arthritis is worse in the mornings then it may help to start work slightly later than usual).
- Job sharing.
- If you are finding a particular aspect of your job is difficult, ask about retraining within your company.
- Talk to someone at work about your concerns. Your company may even have a dedicated occupational health therapist who will be able to help you.
- Request a workplace assessment. This could be arranged through the **Occupational Health Department** of the company or through the **Employment Service's Disability Service Team.**
- Try to stay positive and don't make any hasty decisions regarding your work situation.

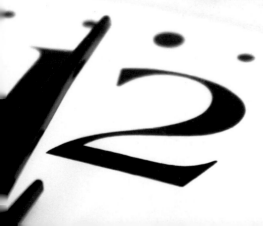

ARTHRITIS AND GETTING AROUND

Staying independent is an important part of coping with arthritis and being able to get around by yourself is an integral part of this. There is no reason why having arthritis should stop you using public transport. Some local authorities run transport schemes to help disabled people get around. These include services like wheelchair-accessible buses, trains and minicabs.

Contact your local authority (listed in the phone book) or your local Disability Information and Advice Line (DIAL UK helpline: 01302 310123) for more details.

The Mobility Advice and Vehicle Information Service (MAVIS)

MAVIS gives practical advice to disabled and older motorists on driving, vehicle adaptation and suitable vehicle types. It will also arrange for you to test drive specially modified vehicles. If you are learning to drive with a disability like arthritis, MAVIS can also put you in touch with specialist driving instructors.

The Motability scheme

The Motability Scheme was established to provide disabled people with safe, reliable and affordable cars. Cars account for 99% of the scheme's activities, with powered wheelchairs and scooters making up the balance (*www.motability.co.uk*).

DRIVING WITH ARTHRITIS

The law dictates that if you have had arthritis that has affected your ability to drive for more than 3 months, you should inform the Drivers Medical Group at the Driver and Vehicle Licensing Agency (DVLA) in Swansea, as well as your insurance company. This should not affect your right to drive or your insurance premiums. You may also qualify for a blue parking badge that will help you to find a parking space closer to where you need to be.

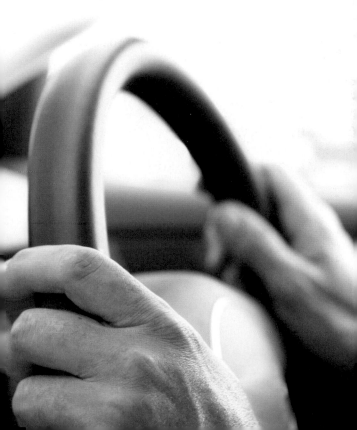

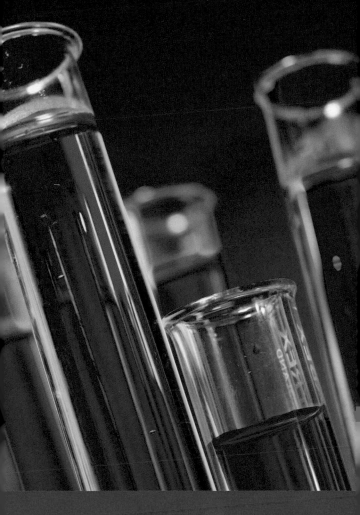

**Simple
science**

SIMPLE SCIENCE

Learning how your joints function and what happens when your arthritis symptoms flare up can help you to understand your condition and make it easier to live with.

We have already seen how arthritis is a disease that causes pain and inflammation in the joints. It doesn't matter which type of arthritis you have been diagnosed with, if it is not managed properly you will usually end up in a certain amount of pain and may have problems getting around and doing certain things. That said, the two major types of arthritis, osteoarthritis and rheumatoid arthritis, are actually quite different in terms of:

- their symptoms

- the rate at which they develop

- the people they affect

- the way in which they are treated.

These differences arise because what's actually going on in the joints is very different. Although both conditions involve the breakdown of cartilage in the joint, osteoarthritis is due to age related changes in which the cartilage becomes thinner in some joints, and the joint becomes less cushioned, whereas rheumatoid arthritis is related to a problem with the body's own immune system.

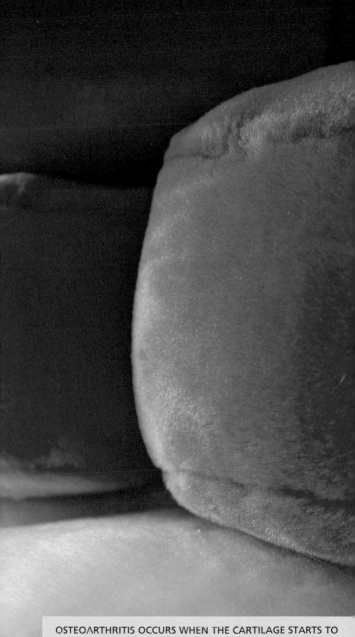

OSTEOARTHRITIS OCCURS WHEN THE CARTILAGE STARTS TO DISAPPEAR AND THE LUBRICATING (SYNOVIAL) FLUID LOSES ITS PROTECTIVE CUSHIONING PROPERTIES.

OSTEOARTHRITIS

Osteoarthritis is also known as *degenerative arthritis*, because the cartilage that protects the bone gradually gets worn away (or degenerates). If the cartilage wears away completely then the ends of the bones can end up rubbing together, which can be extremely painful.

At one stage, scientists believed that osteoarthritis was a natural (and inevitable) consequence of getting older, but we now know this to be untrue. The real story is probably much more complicated. Although it is true that the older you get, the more worn out your joints become, not everyone of a certain age automatically develops arthritis. It is more likely that osteoarthritis can be put down to changes taking place in the microscopic structure of the joints. These changes may start with the cells that make cartilage. The changes that go on in your joint(s) if you have osteoarthritis usually happen in a certain order.

- The cartilage in the joint roughens and becomes worn down (and may disappear altogether).

- Tiny cracks may start to appear in the cartilage.

- Extra bone is laid down to replace the damaged or lost cartilage. The bone underneath the cartilage thickens and grows outwards.

- The amount of bone laid down far exceeds the quantity that is actually needed to replace the damaged cartilage.

- Bony outgrowths (called osteophytes) start to form along the damaged joint.

- Fragments of bone may break off into the joint, which cause the joint to become inflamed and swollen (and painful).

- The synovium starts to produce more synovial fluid than usual, which adds to the swelling in the joint.

- The loss of cartilage, the wearing of bone and the bony outgrowths can all start to change the shape of the joint. This forces the bones out of their normal position and causes deformities.

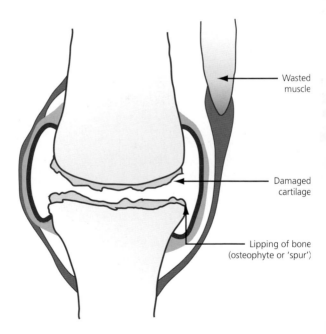

Wasted muscle

Damaged cartilage

Lipping of bone (osteophyte or 'spur')

THE CHANGES THAT OCCUR IN THE JOINTS IN OSTEOARTHRITIS.

RHEUMATOID ARTHRITIS

A case of mistaken identity

Rheumatoid arthritis can be traced back to a malfunction in the immune system. The body produces antibodies that attack the cells of the joint lining (the synovium) because it mistakes it for a foreign invader, making it painful, unstable and deformed. We touched on this 'autoimmunity' briefly in *The basics* section (see page 13).

At the moment, no-one knows exactly what causes them but the more we understand autoimmune diseases, the easier they will be to treat and even prevent. At the moment, however, there are some gaps in what we know.

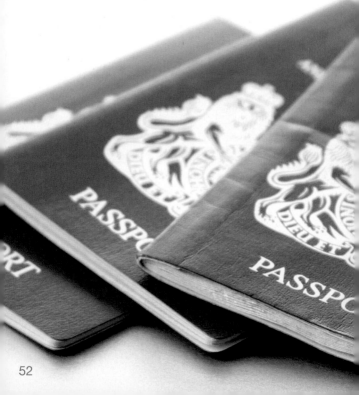

The immune response

So what are antibodies and what do they do?
Antibodies are made by white blood cells called
B-lymphocytes. They can be thought of as
Y-shaped structures, with a special region at the
tip that recognises and attaches to specific foreign
substances, called antigens. Once it has bound to
the antibody, the antigen is neutralised so that it is
no longer harmful. This process is known as the
immune response.

Of course, if the immune response is triggered
inappropriately, perfectly healthy and harmless
cells may become damaged. This is what happens
in the joints when autoantibodies are made in
people with rheumatoid arthritis.

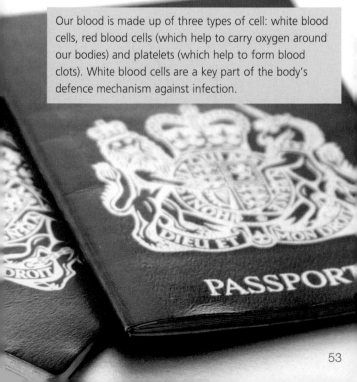

Our blood is made up of three types of cell: white blood
cells, red blood cells (which help to carry oxygen around
our bodies) and platelets (which help to form blood
clots). White blood cells are a key part of the body's
defence mechanism against infection.

How does autoimmunity cause inflammation and pain?

Rheumatoid arthritis usually progresses in three distinct stages.

1. The synovium swells up and becomes inflamed as so-called inflammatory cells in the blood (specialised cells that are responsible for controlling inflammation) flock to the place where they are needed (i.e. the joint). This causes pain, warmth, redness and stiffness.

2. The inflammatory cells in the synovium grow very rapidly, which causes the synovium to thicken and swell further.

3. The inflamed cells then start to break down the bone and cartilage of the joint, often causing the joint to lose its shape and become unstable, painful and unable to move as it once did.

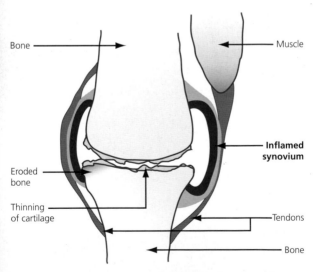

THE CHANGES THAT OCCUR IN THE
JOINTS IN RHEUMATOID ARTHRITIS.

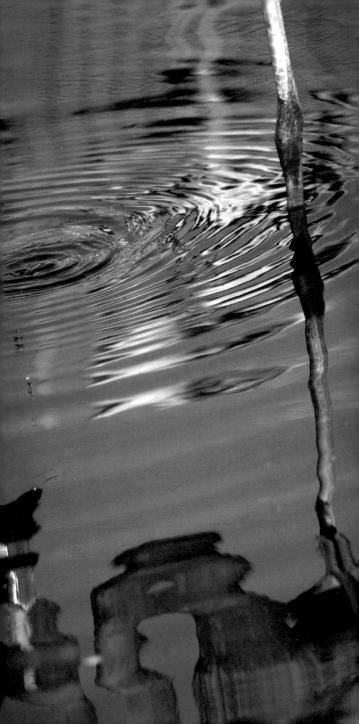

HOW DO WE TREAT ARTHRITIS?

Drugs that treat inflammation

Inflammation is controlled by substances called inflammatory mediators. These substances are made by the body and can make inflammation worse. Prostaglandins are one type of pain-causing inflammatory mediator.

Drugs like aspirin and ibuprofen are called non-steroidal anti-inflammatory drugs (NSAIDs). As their name suggests, they prevent or limit inflammation – specifically by blocking the manufacture of the pain-causing prostaglandins.

Prostaglandins are manufactured in the body by an enzyme called cyclo-oxygenase, or 'COX' for short. The COX enzyme helps to metabolise (or break down) a larger substance called arachidonic acid, into prostaglandins.

So how do the NSAIDs work? By attacking COX and stopping it from doing its job properly, NSAIDs slow down the production of the pain-causing prostaglandins.

However, slowing down the COX enzyme is not always a good thing. Confusingly, there are two forms of the COX enzyme – COX-1 and COX-2. It is mainly the COX-2 variety that is responsible for producing prostaglandins and therefore, blocking COX-2 ultimately helps to relieve pain.

BUT, most NSAIDs block COX-1 as well, which disrupts other biological processes that are far removed from pain transmission. One of these processes is the production of mucus in the stomach, which protects our stomach lining from the damaging stomach acids. This helps to explain why some people develop gastric ulcers, indigestion and general nausea after taking NSAIDs.

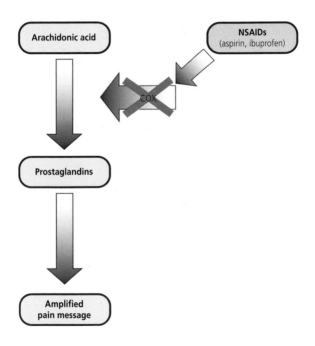

DRUGS THAT CHANGE THE COURSE OF RHEUMATOID ARTHRITIS

These are called disease-modifying antirheumatic drugs (DMARDs) because they can slow down the progress of rheumatoid arthritis and thereby reduce the amount of damage it does to the joints, helping you to stay active for longer. They work in two ways.

1. By reducing inflammation.

2. By altering the activity of the body's immune system.

DMARDs are most useful if they are used as quickly as possible after you have been diagnosed with rheumatoid arthritis. There are many different types of DMARDs, but in the UK, sulphasalazine (Salazopyrin®) and methotrexate (Matrex®) are the ones used most frequently.

Biologic response modifiers

A relatively new group of drugs to emerge as a treatment for rheumatoid arthritis are the biological response modifiers, which include etanercept (Enbrel®), infliximab (Remicade®) and adalimumab (Humira®). These drugs work by blocking the effects of an inflammatory mediator called tumour necrosis factor (TNF) that helps to drive the inflammation process. By stopping TNF from worsening inflammation in the joint, the biological response modifiers can help to slow down the progression of rheumatoid arthritis.

They are still quite new and we do not yet know all the long-term side-effects, so they are usually only used in patients who have tried other DMARDs without success.

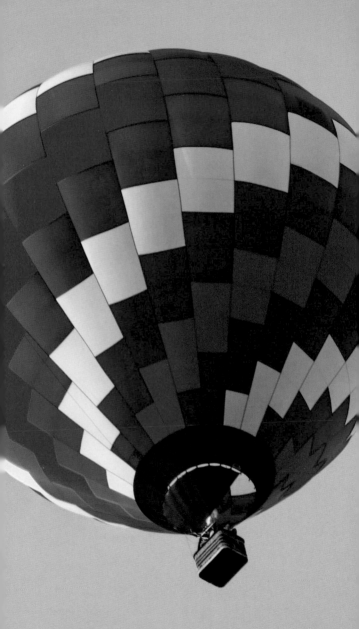

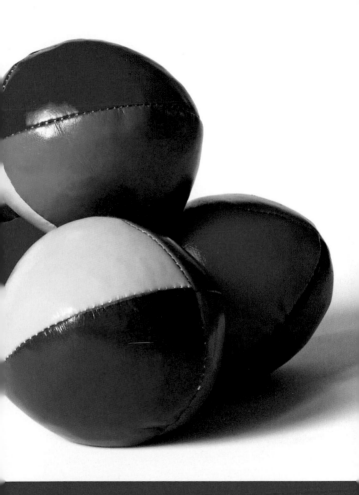

Managing
arthritis

MANAGING ARTHRITIS

Arthritis can be overwhelming and at times it can feel like you will never be able to live a normal life. However, try not to give up hope. Keeping active and staying positive can help you get to grips with your condition.

STAYING IN CONTROL

Most people with arthritis will tell you that there are times when it can feel as though their arthritis is getting the better of them. The trick to handling arthritis is to make sure that these low periods, although sometimes inevitable, are countered by periods of positive thinking. Whilst the loss of function associated with arthritis can sometimes knock your self-confidence and increase your sense of isolation, there is no reason why it should end up controlling your life.

Help yourself cope with your arthritis by:

- using your friends and family for support and encouragement
- asking for help if you need it
- finding out about the many gadgets and services on offer that can help to make your life easier
- finding other people with arthritis and sharing your experiences with them
- using patient forums on the internet to exchange information about arthritis
- taking up new hobbies (or continuing with existing ones wherever possible)
- getting out of the house on a regular basis.

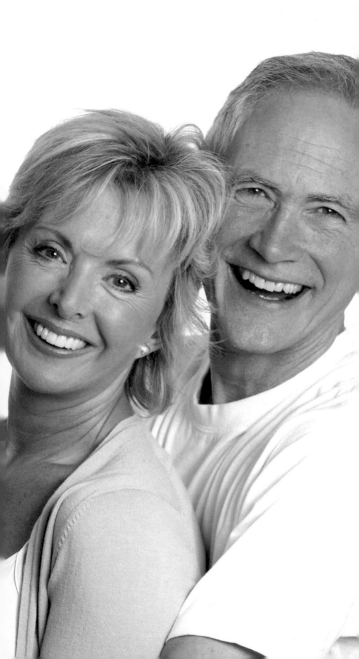

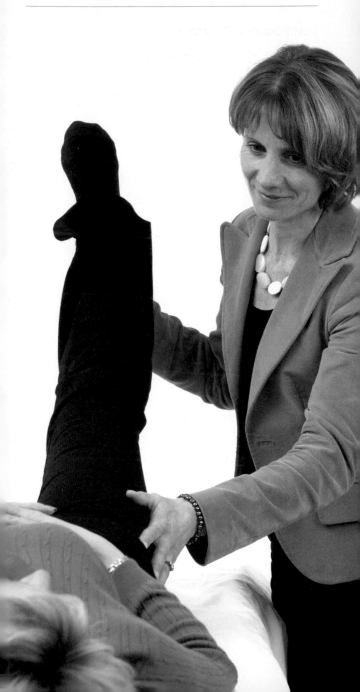

DIAGNOSING ARTHRITIS

For the vast majority of people, your doctor will be able to work out what's wrong with you by:

■ listening to you describe your symptoms

■ examining your joints

■ examining your range of movement

■ looking at your medical history

■ looking at the medical history of your family

■ ordering certain tests (see overleaf).

Putting your symptoms into words can be difficult. It may help you to think about how you would answer the following questions before you visit your doctor.

■ Which of your joints are affected?

■ Have you noticed that your range of movement has changed?

■ Have you started to find it difficult to carry out certain tasks (e.g. buttoning up clothes) that never used to be a problem?

■ Have you experienced any swelling around your joints?

■ How often do you have pain or stiffness?

■ Do your symptoms get worse at certain times of days or after doing certain things?

■ What makes your symptoms better or worse?

Sometimes, your GP may ask you to complete a questionnaire to see to what extent your daily functioning has been compromised. They will use your answers to generate a score, which will tell them to what degree your ability to perform certain tasks has been impaired by your arthritis.

TESTING FOR ARTHRITIS

Although there is no single diagnostic test that can confirm explicitly whether or not you have arthritis (be it osteo- or rheumatoid), there are a number of tests than can help your doctor piece together the evidence. The most common of these are blood tests and scans.

Blood tests

There are a number of reasons why the doctor or the specialist treating you may order a blood test:

■ to help them confirm that you have arthritis

■ to rule out other illnesses

■ to see how advanced your arthritis is

■ to see if your treatment is working.

Blood samples will usually have to be sent away to a laboratory for analysis and so it may take several days for the results to come in. In the laboratory, there are a number of things that can be measured, including:

■ **Rheumatoid factor (RF)**
This is a type of antibody, a special type of blood cell that helps to fight infections. Rheumatoid factor can sometimes be used to show whether or not you have rheumatoid arthritis. The test is not 100% accurate, however, and should only be used to diagnose rheumatoid arthritis together with other pieces of evidence. Some people can have rheumatoid factor in their blood without having rheumatoid arthritis (and *vice versa*).

■ **Full blood count (FBC)**
This measures the levels of a whole host of cells and substances in your bloodstream. It can reveal anaemia or a high white cell count. Both of these are usually just part of the disease and inflammation of rheumatoid arthritis, but sometimes anaemia can be due to lack of iron and a high white count may indicate infection.

■ **Erythrocyte sedimentation rate (ESR)**
This test measures how quickly your red blood cells (erythrocytes) settle down when they are spun around and then left to stand. The ESR is a means of measuring how much inflammation your arthritis is currently causing. Other tests which measure the amount of inflammation include the **plasma viscosity** and the C-related protein (CRP) tests.

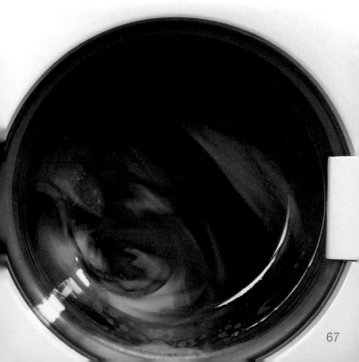

X-rays

X-rays can sometimes be used to identify arthritis. However, because they only detect bones, X-rays do not always show up damage to the joints caused by arthritis and you should not be disappointed if your doctor does not always recommend that you undergo an X-ray (or scan). As a disease like osteoarthritis progresses, the damage to the bone can become more pronounced, and it is at this stage that X-rays are most useful.

CT and MRI scans

CT (computed tomography) and MRI (magnetic resonance imaging) scans are relatively quick and easy ways of obtaining detailed images of the inside of the body, without having to perform surgery.

During a CT scan, X-rays are passed through the body at various angles. As they leave the body, the X-rays are detected by a scanner which uses the information to produce a two-dimensional image of the internal structures of the body, including the joints. CT scanners are gradually being replaced by MRI scanners, which use radio waves (which are safer than X-rays) and high-powered magnetic fields to create two- or three-dimensional images. MRI scanners in particular can distinguish between bone and soft tissue and therefore provide a more detailed picture of the state of a joint as a whole (and not just the bone).

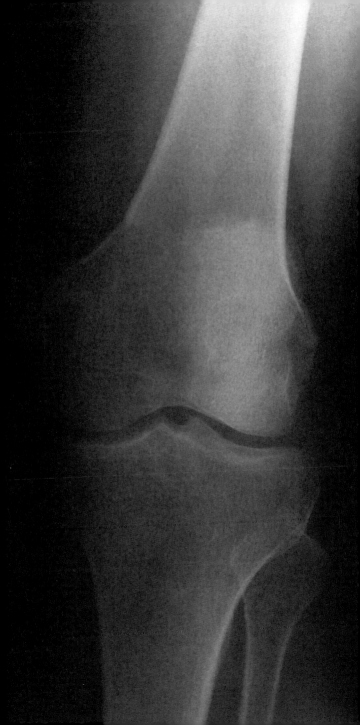

TRUSTING YOUR DOCTOR

Despite the time constraints imposed on doctors these days, your GP should be able to set aside adequate time for you to discuss your symptoms in some depth. He or she should also listen closely to what you're saying and give you a satisfactory explanation for what you are experiencing and reassure you insofar as is possible. Although you may not like what your doctor is telling you, trust their experience and judgment. Try to work with them. Having said that, if your doctor is not sympathetic to your concerns, then try another doctor. This is after all your right.

Will I be referred?

Although many people with arthritis can be managed at their local doctor's surgery, your GP may sometimes choose to refer you to an arthritis specialist at a hospital – usually a consultant rheumatologist or an orthopaedic surgeon (if he thinks that an operation may help you).

Sometimes you may be referred on the basis of the results of the tests that your doctor has ordered for you, or if the course of treatment that your doctor has recommended does not appear to be improving your symptoms. You will usually be seen as an outpatient at your local hospital. Many of the tests outlined above (like X-rays and MRI scans) will be carried out in a hospital setting.

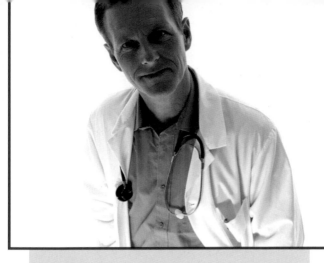

SPECIALIST

If your arthritis is proving difficult to diagnose or control, or is particularly advanced, your GP may feel that you will benefit from my particular experience in looking after people with arthritis and so refer you to me.

I am a hospital-based doctor specially trained to manage conditions affecting the joints. Depending on the type of arthritis I specialise in, I may sometimes be known as an orthopaedic surgeon (osteoarthritis) or a rheumatologist (rheumatoid arthritis). If you have any kind of bone-related surgery (like a hip or knee replacement, for example), as a specialist orthopaedic surgeon, I will be responsible for carrying out the procedure. If you have been diagnosed with rheumatoid arthritis and require treatment with disease-modifying drugs (DMARDs), as a rheumatologist, I will be the one who initiates your treatment and monitors your progress.

How is arthritis treated?

Once you have been diagnosed with arthritis, your doctor (or specialist) will set out the most appropriate course of treatment for you. Try to take as active a role as possible in the management programme your doctor devises. Ask lots of questions during your consultations – remember this is YOUR time. The more you learn about arthritis, the easier it will be to manage. Gather and read as much information about arthritis as you can.

The way in which your arthritis is treated will depend on the type of arthritis that you have. However, the overall aims of any treatment programme are to:

■ reduce or relieve pain

■ reduce inflammation

■ improve your mobility

■ improve your quality of life.

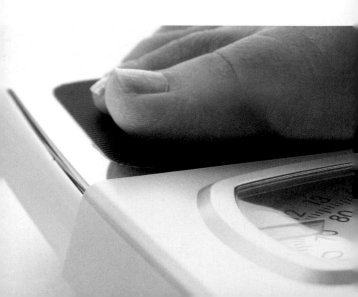

What can I do to help myself?

If you have been diagnosed with arthritis, your doctor will probably recommend that you make certain changes to your lifestyle. These may include:

- changing certain aspects of your diet

- losing weight (if you are overweight)

- exercising on a regular basis.

These changes are all things you can do yourself. As well as helping you to control your arthritis, these changes will also help to improve your general health, which after all, can't be a bad thing! However, always talk to your doctor before introducing any lifestyle change.

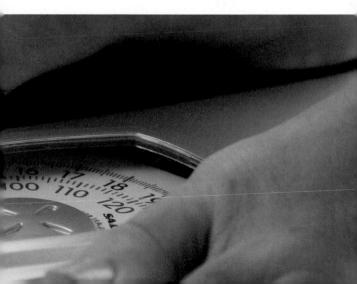

DIET AND ARTHRITIS

The best way of making sure that the food you eat is keeping your joints healthy, is to follow a balanced diet. This will also help to control your weight, and losing excess weight can help to relieve some of the pressure that your joints are under. Of course, eating healthily is also good for your general health and can help to reduce your risk of developing heart disease (for example, by lowering your cholesterol) and can even help to protect you against certain types of cancer.

Eating a healthy, balanced diet involves:

- eating fruit and vegetables on a daily basis
- eating fish at least once a week (especially oily fish like mackerel, sardines, salmon and herring)
- replacing saturated fat (found in butter, cream, fatty meats and pastries) with mono- or polyunsaturated fats and oils (found in fish oils and plant seed oils)
- eating less sugar
- eating more fibre (found in wholegrain starchy foods and beans, peas and lentils)
- cutting down on salt and salty foods and looking out for hidden salt in processed foods
- eating plenty of calcium- and iron-rich foods.

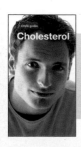

For more information see
Cholesterol

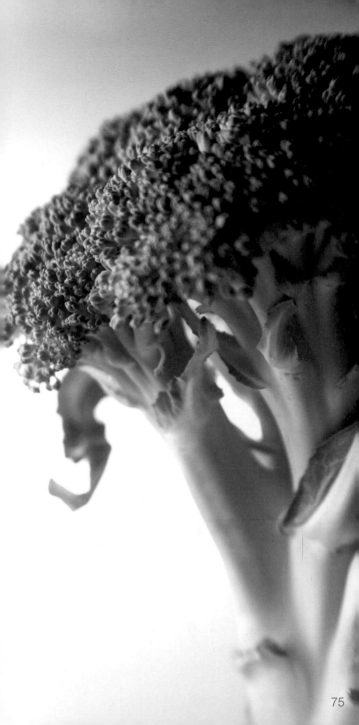

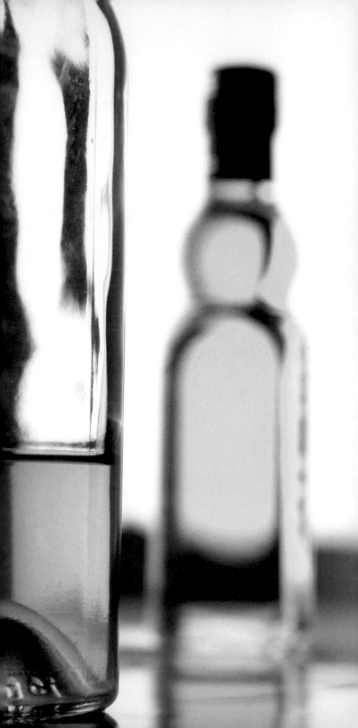

Oils and arthritis

There is some evidence that consuming certain types of oil can help to improve symptoms in some people with arthritis (this is currently an area under intense investigation). Bear in mind that these oils will not stop joint damage progressing, but they may improve your symptoms. The oils in question are those that contain something called essential fatty acids (EFAs), substances that the body cannot make itself and must acquire from the outside world. There are two types of EFAs – omega-3 and omega-6 oils.

- Omega-3 oils are found in oily fish like herring, mackerel, pilchards, sardines and salmon.

- Omega-6 oils are derived from plants (e.g. rapeseed oil, linseed oil, soya oil and walnuts).

Gout and food

Gout is a type of arthritis that arises when uric acid (the chief waste product in urine) builds up in the blood and accumulates in the joints. Most uric acid comes from the breakdown of substances called purines in the body itself. Small amounts are contained in certain foods.

If you have gout then you may find that avoiding foods that contain a lot of purines may help, for example liver, heart, kidney, meat extract (e.g. Oxo™), anchovies, crab, herring, mackerel, sardines, and shrimps, but this is usually only a factor if you have an unusual diet that includes large quantities of these foods. Alcohol, on the other hand, is best avoided if possible as this definitely makes gout worse.

Exclusion diets

Some people find that some symptoms of arthritis can be aggravated by specific foods. If this is the case, it may make sense to rule them out of your diet. This is usually done by cutting out the foods that you think may be aggravating your symptoms to see if they improve, and then gradually reintroducing them to see whether your symptoms come back. If symptoms return then it is possible that this type of food is making your rheumatoid arthritis worse and it may help to avoid it in the future.

Exclusion (or elimination) diets are not always advisable and do not help everyone. Be careful that you don't end up ruling out too many different foods to the extent that your diet or eating habits are drastically compromised or you are losing out on essential nutrients. Strict exclusion diets have very low success rates and can often do more harm than good.

If you do make changes to your diet make sure that you do it gradually so that your body has time to adjust. Also make sure that you seek advice from your GP before embarking on anything too drastic.

WEIGHT LOSS

There are many reasons why we are less active than we used to be. Cars, televisions and computers may make our lives easier, but they may also be causing us some significant health problems. By becoming less active (as well as eating more 'junk' food) we are becoming heavier (and in many cases obese). As a consequence, we are putting more pressure on our joints. Maintaining an ideal body weight (for example by using the BMI calculator below) can help to improve arthritis by reducing the stresses our joints and bones are under.

CALCULATE YOUR OWN BODY MASS INDEX (BMI)

It's very simple to work out your own BMI, to see whether your weight has put you at risk of arthritis. Grab a tape measure, a set of bathroom scales and a calculator and follow these two steps.

▪ Measure your height in metres. Multiply this number by itself and write down the answer, for example:

$$1.80 \text{ (metres)} \times 1.80 = 3.24$$

▪ Measure your weight in kilograms. Divide it by the number you wrote down in the first step, for example:

$$80 \text{ (kilograms)} \div 3.24 = 24.7$$

The number you get is your BMI. As a general rule, for adults aged over 20, the BMI relates to the following:

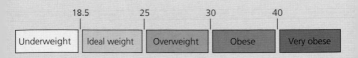

	18.5	25	30	40
Underweight	Ideal weight	Overweight	Obese	Very obese

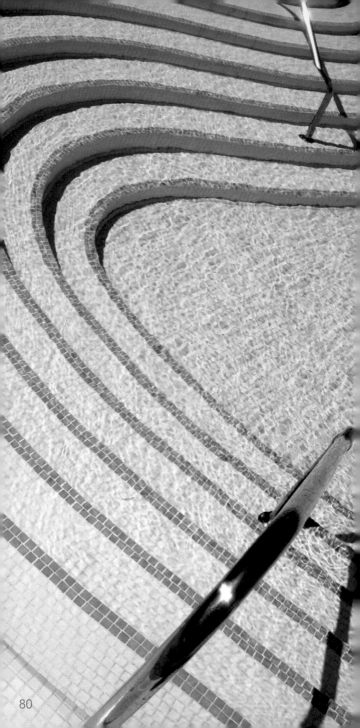

ARTHRITIS AND EXERCISE

You should not assume that you can't exercise just because you have arthritis. Many people with arthritis can experience some relief from their symptoms by taking regular exercise. However, it is vitally important that you balance the amount of exercise you do with enough rest periods in between. Do not overdo it and never exercise during periods when your symptoms are flaring-up. Always seek medical advice before taking up any new type of exercise.

- Exercise helps you to stay in shape, and staying in shape (and in particular losing weight) can help to take pressure off your joints.

- Lifting weights will help to build up your muscle strength.

- Exercise helps to keep you active and mobile and gets you out of the house.

- Exercising is a good way of taking your mind off your arthritis.

Good and bad exercise

Although regular exercise is proven to benefit people with arthritis, doing the wrong type of exercise can sometimes make your symptoms worse. This is why it is so important that you seek advice before embarking on any programme of exercise. Ask your GP, a physiotherapist or a qualified gym instructor what kind of exercise is most appropriate for you. If an exercise hurts or feels uncomfortable, you should stop doing it immediately.

Aerobic exercise

This is exercise that raises your heart rate and thereby helps to control your weight and builds up your stamina. The best forms of aerobic exercise for people with arthritis are walking, cycling, and swimming. Even doing the vacuuming or mowing the lawn can get the heart pumping faster! Swimming is particularly good because it gets your heart going and builds up your muscle strength, but because the water is cushioning your body, the strain that your joints are under is very much reduced.

Range of movement exercises

These are exercises that repeatedly bend and straighten a joint within its non-painful range. This may be as simple as swinging your legs as you sit on a chair or as active as going for a gentle bike ride. Putting your joints through their full range of movement on a regular basis (i.e. every day) can help to preserve your range of movement and keep your joints flexible. However, you should never try to push your joints further than they can go naturally.

Strengthening exercises

These exercises help to strengthen the muscles that move, support and protect your joints. Of course, no-one is suggesting that you start weightlifting, but simply tightening and releasing your muscles on a regular basis can help to keep your muscles strong and keep you mobile. Gradually build up the intensity of the exercise, perhaps by holding cans of food or bags of sugar as you exercise.

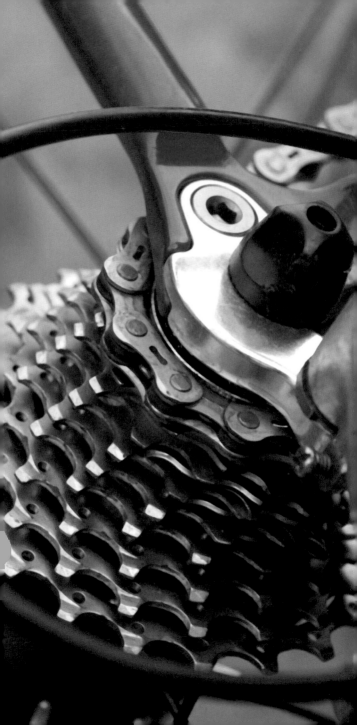

Arthritis and footwear

We have over 30 joints in each foot, and many of these can be affected by arthritis (the big toe in particular). It's not just the joints of the feet that may be affected. Tendons and other soft tissue areas can also become inflamed and tender. Bunions (bony lumps that develop on the side of the foot at the base of the big toe) can be extremely painful if they are not managed properly. It is therefore very important that you take good care of your feet if you suffer from arthritis. This may mean:

- wearing comfortable air-cushioned shoes (e.g. Hoto™, Ecco™, Clarks™)

- making sure your shoes fit properly when you buy them

- wearing arch support

- wearing padding to protect lumps and bumps on your feet (bunion pads)

- using a pumice stone to get rid of the build up of hard skin

- checking your feet every day for problems

- washing your feet every day in warm, soapy water

- changing your socks every day

- trying not to stand for long periods (to take pressure off your feet)

- trimming your toe nails regularly.

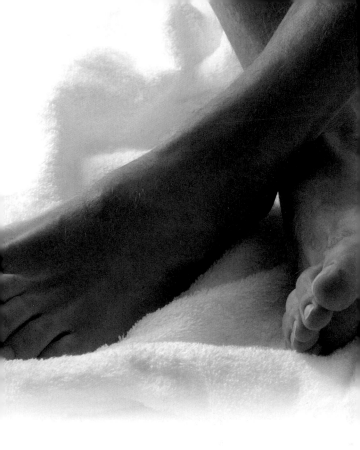

Podiatry and arthritis

A podiatrist is a person who specialises in the care and treatment of feet. Although, it is possible to see a podiatrist on the NHS, you will usually need a referral from your GP. For speed and convenience, many people cover the costs of the treatment themselves. Always seek advice from a specialist before using foot treatments like bunion pads, pumice stones or abrasive boards.

TREATING ARTHRITIS WITH DRUGS

The treatment of arthritis usually (but not always) takes the form of some kind of drug treatment. This may be simple painkillers (analgesics) or specialist drugs that can help to change the course of the disease (for rheumatoid arthritis only). The type of drug treatment you will be offered depends on the type of arthritis that you have been diagnosed with. In this section, we will look at each disease in turn.

- For osteoarthritis, drug treatment revolves around providing pain relief.
- For rheumatoid arthritis, drugs can be used to relieve pain and reduce inflammation but may also be used to slow down the progression of the disease itself.

The drugs and medications referred to in this Simple Guide are believed to be currently in widespread use in the UK. Medical science can evolve rapidly, but to the best of our knowledge, this is a reasonable reflection of clinical practice at the time of going to press.

Source: British National Formulary.

Pain relief for osteoarthritis

Painkillers – or analgesics – are drugs that work by interfering with the way that pain signals are transmitted through the body. If you are experiencing some degree of pain because of your osteoarthritis, you doctor will probably recommend that you take an analgesic, especially during those periods when your symptoms are flaring up. The strength of the analgesic you are prescribed will depend on how severe your pain is. Initially, your doctor will usually recommend that you take one of the 'milder' analgesics, like paracetamol, aspirin or ibuprofen. These drugs can be obtained from your pharmacist without a prescription.

Many of the painkillers that you can obtain over the counter from your pharmacist are sufficient to control the pain associated with arthritis if they are taken properly. Remember to always ask your pharmacist for advice, never exceed the stated dose and beware of overdosing unwittingly by taking more than one branded product that contains the same active ingredient (for example aspirin or paracetamol).

Of course, if these milder analgesics are not sufficient to control your pain, then you should consult your doctor, who may be able to prescribe you something stronger. When it comes to analgesia, you will usually be offered medications in a certain order according to what has worked (or not worked) for you in the past. The usual hierarchy of pain relief for osteoarthritis is as follows.

1. Paracetamol.

2. Paracetamol plus a low dose of an opioid drug (as Co-codamol® 8/500 or Co-dydramol® 10/500).

3. A low dose of an NSAID (e.g. aspirin or ibuprofen) for a trial period of about 1 month.

4. Paracetamol plus a low dose of an NSAID.

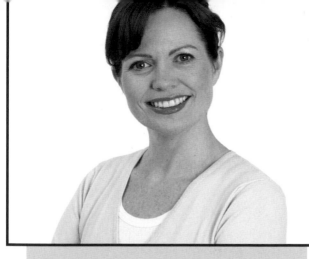

RHEUMATOLOGY NURSE SPECIALIST

I am a specially trained nurse with experience in looking after people with rheumatoid arthritis. Traditionally, I am based in a hospital. You will usually be put in touch with me through your consultant rheumatologist, who will have already diagnosed you as having rheumatoid arthritis and will have decided upon a course of treatment.

Often, I am trained to carry out many of the tasks previously assigned to doctors like joint examinations, reviewing and requesting investigations and performing joint injections. My specialist knowledge and experience allows me to answer any specific questions you may have about any aspect of your rheumatoid arthritis, and explain your treatments to you. I can also liaise with the other members of your care team (e.g. GP and rheumatologist) and can help to arrange and co-ordinate your check-up appointments. I can also offer you support and advice over the phone, should you require it, or should your rheumatoid arthritis prevent you from coming into the clinic.

Paracetamol

Paracetamol and NSAIDs are generally equally effective at relieving pain, but paracetamol is less irritating to the stomach. For this reason, it is often used preferentially in elderly people and in other susceptible groups such as pregnant women, people with asthma or people with gastric ulcers. Overdosing on paracetamol is extremely dangerous because it may cause permanent and irreversible damage to your liver, but if taken according to instructions it is much less likely to cause side-effects than NSAIDs for example.

Always take paracetamol as directed on the packaging (two 500 mg tablets every 4 hours up to a maximum of eight 500 mg tablets in 24 hours) and consult your doctor if your pain persists. You should also be aware that paracetamol can be 'hidden' in some branded products so take extra care not to overdose inadvertently.

Non-steroidal anti-inflammatory drugs (NSAIDs)

As the name suggests, NSAIDs like aspirin and ibuprofen help to relieve pain by reducing the inflammation that is causing it. They are amongst the most widely used types of pain relief. But there is a catch. The major problem associated with NSAIDs is the irritation they cause to the stomach

and digestive system (see *Simple science* page 56).
Taking these drugs after eating can help to
prevent this, but as a general rule, NSAIDs are
not suitable for:

■ people over 65 years of age

■ people with a history of gastric ulcers

■ people using blood-thinning drugs
like warfarin

■ people with some other diseases like heart
disease, kidney disease, diabetes and asthma.

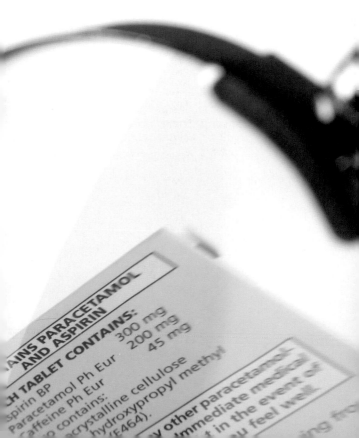

The cyclo-oxygenase-2 (COX-2) inhibitors

The COX-2 inhibitors (e.g. celecoxib [Celebrex®], etodolac [Eccoxolac®], etoricoxib [Arcoxia®] and meloxicam [Mobic®]) are NSAIDs that are used to relieve the joint pain associated with arthritis. In theory, these drugs do not disrupt the stomach and digestive systems as much as the conventional NSAIDs (see *Simple science* page 56) and this is seen as a major advantage for those people who have to take them on a regular basis.

Recently, however, evidence has emerged to suggest that some types of COX-2 inhibitors (e.g. celecoxib [Celebrex®] and valdecoxib [Bextra®]) may increase the likelihood of cardiovascular complications (like heart attacks) in some people. Therefore as a precaution, it is recommended that these drugs should only be used in people who are particularly susceptible to the gastrointestinal side-effects of standard NSAIDs, and only after their risk of heart complications has been evaluated and shown to be low. At this time, the availability of the COX-2

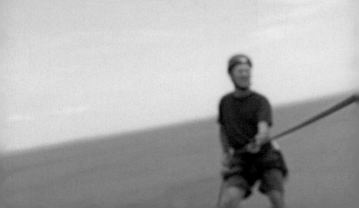

inhibitors is constantly changing in line with extensive investigations into their safety. This will influence whether or not your doctor can prescribe you these drugs. If you are currently taking any of these drugs and have concerns, you should contact your GP.

Very recent evidence suggests that not just the COX-2 inhibitors but all NSAIDs (including ibuprofen and naproxen) can be linked to an increased risk of having a heart attack. It should be remembered that this is only preliminary data and further investigation into these drugs is needed before any firm conclusions can be reached. In the meantime, the Medicines and Healthcare Products Regulatory Agency (MHRA) advises patients to use the lowest effective dose of NSAID for the shortest time necessary.

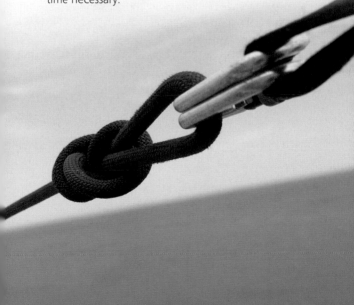

Compound analgesics

If after a while you find that paracetamol alone is not providing you with adequate pain relief, it may be worth trying a compound analgesic. This is a drug that contains a mixture of two analgesics, usually paracetamol and another type of analgesic, like codeine. Co-codamol® (which combines paracetamol with codeine) is an example of a compound analgesic. You will need to be prescribed this by your doctor.

Co-proxamol®, a compound analgesic containing paracetamol and dextropropoxyphene (a pain-killing drug that is similar in structure to the opioid methadone) was until recently used by many people suffering from the chronic pain associated with arthritis. However, from 2005 Co-proxamol® is being withdrawn from general use because of concerns that it is too dangerous if taken in large quantities.

Drugs often have more than one name. A generic name, which refers to its active ingredient, and a brand name, which is the registered trade name given to it by the pharmaceutical company. Ibuprofen is a generic name and Nurofen® is a brand name.

THE TYPES OF ANALGESIC THAT MAY BE USED TO RELIEVE THE PAIN ASSOCIATED WITH ARTHRITIS

Drug	Brand names
Over-the-counter (OTC)	
Paracetamol	Calpol®, Disprol®, Hedex®, Panadol®
Aspirin	Alka-Seltzer®, Anadin®, Disprin®
Ibuprofen	Advil®, Cuprofen®, Nurofen®
Compound analgesics:	
– Paracetamol and codeine	Solpadeine Max®, Ultramol®, Panadol Ultra®
– Aspirin and codeine	Codis 500®
– Ibuprofen and codeine	Nurofen® Plus, Solpaflex®
Prescription-only medicines (POM)	
Aspirin	Caprin®
Ibuprofen	Arthrofen®, Brufen®, Ebufac®
Naproxen	Arthroxen®, Naprosyn®, Synflex®
Diclofenac sodium	Acoflam®, Defenac®, Dicloflex®, Volraman®, Voltarol®
Compound analgesics:	
– Paracetamol and codeine	Co-codamol®, Tylex®
– Ibuprofen and codeine	Codafen Continus®
– Aspirin and codeine	Co-codaprin®

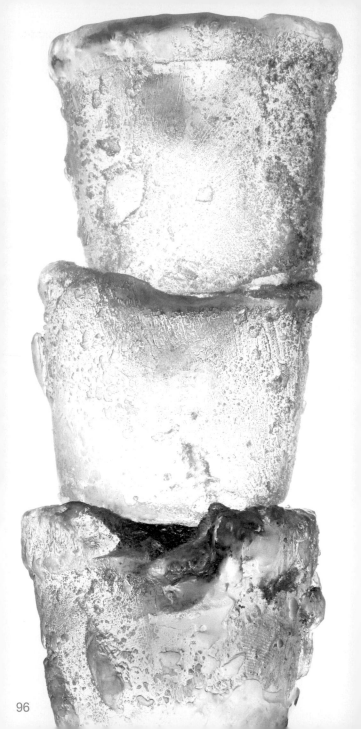

OPTIONAL EXTRAS

In addition to the 'conventional' forms of analgesia mentioned previously, your doctor may recommend that you try one of the following.

■ A gel, cream or spray. This may contain something that warms or soothes the joints (e.g. Cuprofen®, Deep Heat®, Radian® and Ralgex Cream®) or it may contain either an NSAID (like ibuprofen) or a substance extracted from chilli peppers called capsaicin.

■ Injection of a corticosteroid into the knee or the base of the thumb. This can temporarily relieve pain in the joint and must be carried out by a qualified healthcare professional. Usually injections are limited to a maximum of about one every 3 or 4 months.

The drug treatment of rheumatoid arthritis

Rheumatoid arthritis is treated in a different way to osteoarthritis. Although you may still be prescribed analgesics to relieve the pain that is associated with joint inflammation, there are also a number of other types of medication that can be used to slow down the rate at which the disease progresses. If you have rheumatoid arthritis, your doctor will probably prescribe you a combination of:

- simple analgesics

- NSAIDs

- disease-modifying antirheumatic drugs (DMARDs).

NSAIDs and rheumatoid arthritis

People with rheumatoid arthritis will usually need to take NSAIDs on a long-term basis, rather than just during those periods when their symptoms are particularly bad (as may be the case for osteoarthritis). Bearing in mind the stomach irritation that can be associated with NSAIDs (see *Simple science* page 56), it is important that your doctor gives you the lowest dose that is necessary to control your symptoms. This will limit your chances of developing gastric irritation. Older people or those with a history of ulcers may be offered a drug called a proton pump inhibitor to further reduce their risk (e.g. omeprazole [Losec®], esomeprazole [Nexium®], lansoprazole [Zoton®], pantoprazole [Protium®] and rabeprazole [Pariet®]).

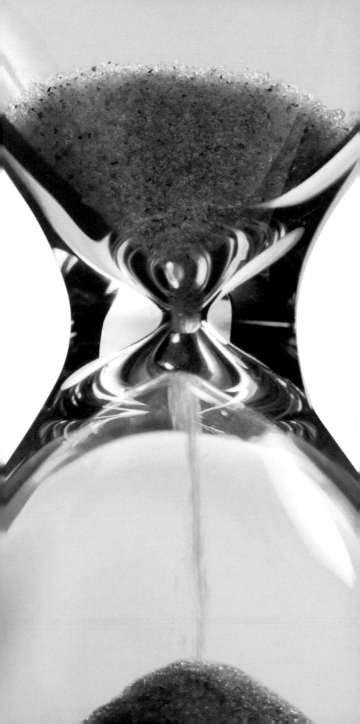

Disease-modifying antirheumatic drugs (DMARDs)

Soon after you are diagnosed with rheumatoid arthritis, you will usually be treated with a DMARD. This will help to control your symptoms and may delay the rate at which the disease can progress, hence the term disease-modifying. If you are prescribed a DMARD, your treatment will usually be managed by a specialist.

DMARDs may take several weeks to start working, but once they do, it may be possible to gradually lower the dose of NSAID you are taking. If you get on well with them, you will usually continue to receive a DMARD for as long as it provides you with some kind of relief from your symptoms.

There are many different types of DMARDs, but in the UK, sulphasalazine (Salazopyrin®) and methotrexate (Matrex®) are the ones used most frequently. Other types include gold, D-penicillamine, azathioprine (Imuran®), cyclophosphamide, ciclosporin and leflunomide (Arava®). DMARDs are given as tablets, with the exception of gold, which can be given as an injection into muscle or buttocks (sodium aurothiomalate [Myocrisin®]). Unfortunately, like most drugs, DMARDs can be associated with side-effects, and these may include skin rashes, diarrhoea, nausea and vomiting, headache and hair loss. Rarely, they can affect the eyes, liver and the kidneys so your doctor or specialist may want to monitor the functioning of these organs with regular blood tests (usually monthly) as your treatment goes on.

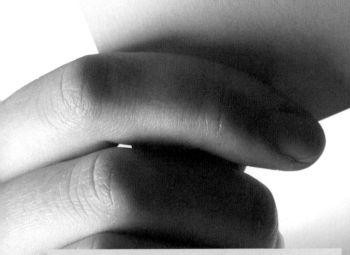

No drug treatment is without side-effects, and different people may respond in slightly different ways to the same medicine. If you experience symptoms which you think may be due to the medication you are taking, you should talk to your doctor, pharmacist or nurse. If the side-effect is unusual or severe, your GP may decide to report it to the MHRA. The MHRA operates a 'Yellow Card Scheme' which is designed to flag up potentially dangerous drug effects and thereby protect your safety. The procedure has changed recently to allow patients to report adverse drug reactions themselves. Visit *www.yellowcard.gov.uk* for more information. You should always ask your doctor if you are concerned about any aspect of your arthritis management plan.

Biological response modifiers

The biological response modifiers (e.g. etanercept [Enbrel®], infliximab [Remicade®] and adalimumab [Humira®]) are currently reserved for people who have tried the traditional DMARDs and have failed to respond to them. Scientists are still investigating the long-term effects of these drugs and so we can expect to learn more about the way they work and how effective they are in the future.

The treatment of osteoporosis

The drugs available for treating osteoporosis work by balancing the rate at which old bone is broken down with the rate at which new bone is made. There is a growing range of drugs available to your doctor for treating osteoporosis:

- bisphosphonates (e.g. alendronic acid [Fosamax®], risedronate sodium [Actonel®])

- dual-action bone agents (strontium ranelate [Protelos®])

- selective oestrogen receptor modulators (abbreviated to SERMs; e.g. raloxifene hydrochloride [Evista®])

- parathyroid hormone (e.g. teriparatide [Forsteo®])

- calcitriol (Rocaltrol®, Calcijex®)

- calcitonin (Miacalcic®)

- hormone replacement therapy (HRT).

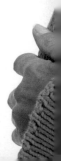

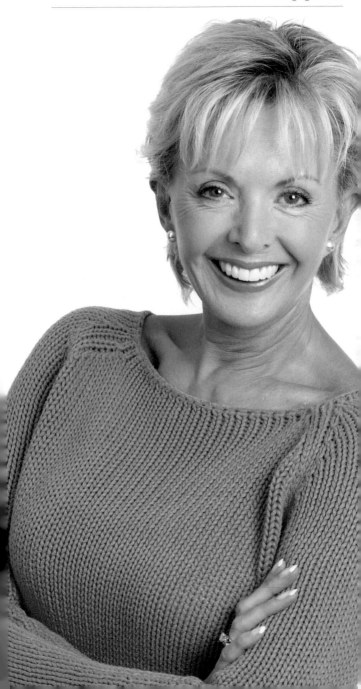

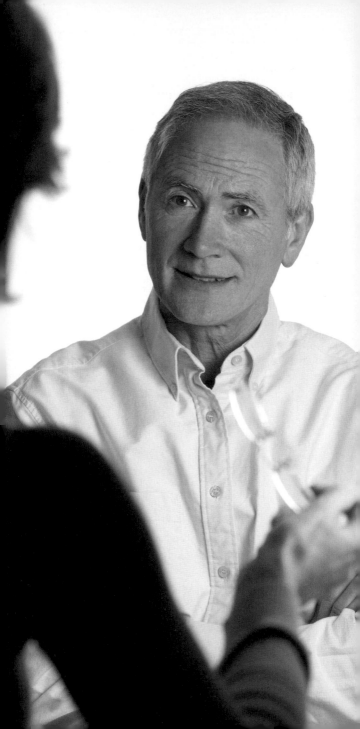

SURGERY

Although most people with arthritis will never need surgery, it can be used as a last resort if all other treatment options have failed to work or if the joint is very badly damaged. As arthritis medications become more sophisticated, the number of people having surgery is falling. For those people who do qualify for surgery, it can relieve pain, improve mobility and reduce stiffness.

No surgical procedure is without its risks and it is important that you understand what your specialist is proposing to do before you give your consent – make sure that you ask plenty of questions like:

- what are the risks associated with this procedure?
- how long have you been doing this procedure and how many do you do in a year?
- how long will I have to remain in hospital?
- how much time will I need to take off work?
- will I still have to take medication even after the operation?

Going private

Unfortunately, due to sheer demand, the NHS waiting lists for joint surgery can be very long (for more information try the NHS National Waiting List helpline – 0208 9831133). For this reason, many people choose to 'go private' and fund their operation themselves or using a private health insurance policy. Although private treatment can be much quicker and allows you to choose when and where you have your operation, it can be hugely expensive. For example, the average hip replacement costs between £7,000 and £10,000.

Joint replacement

This procedure involves the partial or total replacement of the affected joint (usually the hips, knee or shoulder, but sometimes the hand, elbow or ankle). During the operation, the surgeon will remove the damaged joint and replace it with an artificial one (made from plastic, ceramics or metal). Joint replacements usually last between 10 and 15 years, but this will depend on what it is made from. Because the replacements do not last forever, it is usually better to wait for a few years before you have a joint replacement. Around 40,000 hip and knee operations and 4,000–5,000 shoulder operations take place in the UK every year.

Hip resurfacing

Resurfacing the damaged joint is a less drastic alternative to replacing the joint completely, and is most usually performed in younger people with arthritis. Typically, the surface of the joint (usually the hip joint) is replaced by a metal hemisphere and the joint socket is lined with a metal shell. This ensures that as much of the original bone is kept as possible, the idea being that this method will be more durable than a total joint replacement. The procedure is still in its infancy and will continue to develop over the coming years.

RESURFACING HIP JOINTS CAN HELP TO PRESERVE JOINT FUNCTION.

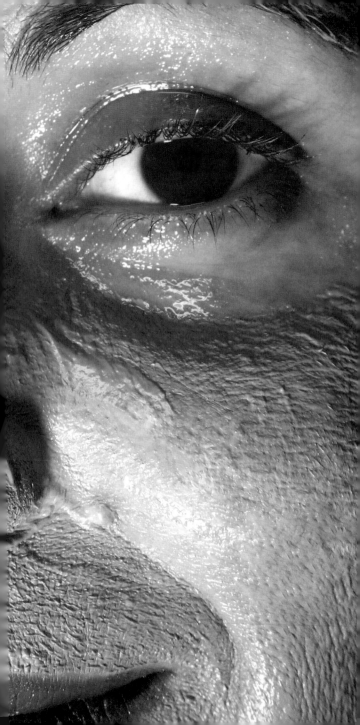

Physiotherapy

Physiotherapy uses physical means (such as massage, exercise, heat or electricity) to maintain and restore your physical and mental well-being. It is an active rather than a passive treatment and is usually concerned with keeping your joints moving and maintaining muscle strength. As well as relieving the pain that is associated with arthritis, physiotherapy can also be used to treat a large number of other common ailments like muscle sprains, sports injuries, incontinence, osteoporosis, depression and asthma.

You may be referred to a physiotherapist by your doctor, or you may choose to see one independently. Whether you see a practitioner privately or through the NHS, the standard of care you will receive is exactly the same. However, if you are willing to pay for the treatment yourself, it may be that you get seen faster than you would if you waited to go through the NHS. If you choose to approach a physiotherapist directly and pay for your treatment, fees range from £25 to £50 for a single session.

Hydrotherapy

Your local hospital may offer hydrotherapy courses (although you will need a referral from your doctor). The hydrotherapy pool is heated to a high temperature (rather like that of a bath) and this can help to relax joints and ease pain.

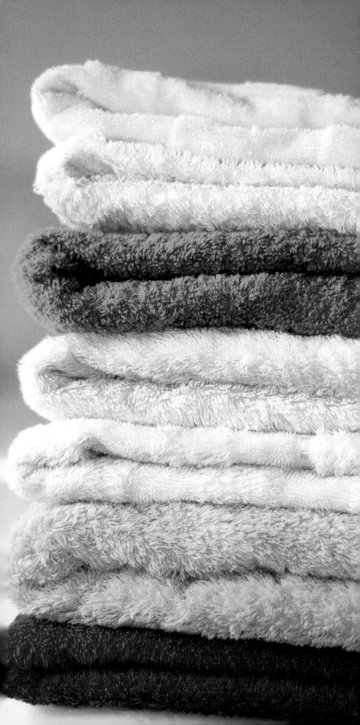

Social security benefits

You and the people who care for you may be entitled to certain benefits and services which can help you with the day-to-day costs and difficulties of living with arthritis.

If you have problems getting around or coping with things like getting dressed or washing because of your arthritis, you may be entitled to a **Disability Living Allowance** (if you are under 65) or an **Attendance Allowance** (if you are over 65). If the person who cares for you is aged over 16 and regularly spends at least 35 hours a week looking after you, they may be entitled to a **Carer's Allowance**. The Citizens Advice Bureau (*www.citizensadvice.org.uk*) or your local county council can help you to complete the forms to apply for these benefits.

There are various other organisations that may be able to help you to find out whether you are entitled to help. The contact details of some of these are listed at the end of this book (see *Simple extras* page 128). In addition to medical care services, such as home-based treatment from a physiotherapist, you may be entitled to practical help, in the form of home-delivered meals, for example, although these services are unlikely to be offered free of charge.

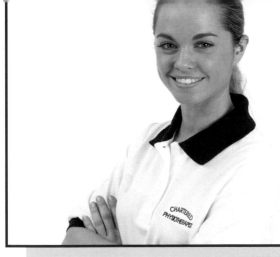

PHYSIOTHERAPIST

You may be referred to me by your GP or your specialist at any time, be it when you are first diagnosed or later on when your arthritis is at a more advanced stage.

At your first appointment I will usually ask you questions about your symptoms and any difficulties you are experiencing with your movement, getting around and performing daily activities. I can then give you information about how to protect your joints and how to manage those periods when your symptoms flare up. I will also be able to teach you a range of simple exercises that will help to strengthen your bones and muscles, increase your range of movement, improve your balance and help you to preserve your functioning. I will look at the way in which you walk and can recommend ways in which you can improve your posture (e.g. using walking aids or specially adapted footwear). If it is appropriate, I can refer you on to see a foot care specialist, called a podiatrist.

Exercises done in water (hydrotherapy) can be particularly useful for relieving the joint pain associated with arthritis and I can arrange for you to take part in these sessions (usually held at your local hospital).

Complementary therapies for arthritis

In addition to the treatments we have already looked at that are available for managing arthritis, the condition also lends itself to a number of 'complementary therapies'. These treatment options, as suggested by their name, are designed to complement the more conventional treatments, not to replace them. It is wise to be cautious about whether a particular treatment is worthwhile and safe for you, given your symptoms and your medical history. If you are considering trying one, talk to your doctor (who may be able to refer you to an NHS practitioner or recommend a reputable private one).

Acupuncture

Acupuncture is an ancient Chinese medical treatment that involves the insertion of very fine needles into the body at specific points. There are around 500 acupuncture points all over the body. By mapping 'energy pathways' throughout the body, acupuncture affects the way certain organs work.

At your first consultation, an acupuncturist will ask you about your symptoms, your medical history and your health in general. They may also feel the quality, rhythm and strength of the pulses on both of your wrists. It is important that you choose an acupuncturist who is suitably qualified. The British Acupuncture Council (*www.acupuncture.org.uk*) will be able to advise you. Because arthritis is a long-term condition and persists over long periods of time, you may require regularly scheduled treatments over several months.

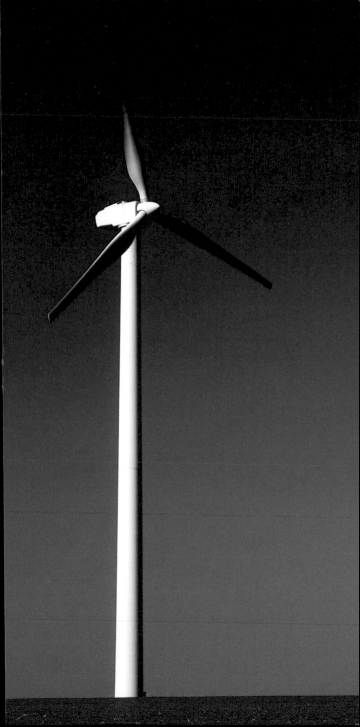

Transcutaneous electrical nerve stimulation (TENS)

TENS is a technique that cleverly interrupts the 'I hurt' messages that are being sent to your brain from a damaged joint. If these messages, which travel along nerves, do not reach the brain, you do not feel the pain. TENS also stimulates the brain to produce 'pain-killing hormones' called endorphins. The TENS machine is about the size of a personal stereo, and can be clipped to clothing in a similar manner. It has electrode pads which you need to stick to the skin, and although you might feel some tingling while the machine is working, this should not be painful or unpleasant. TENS does not work for everyone, and it should not be used at all in some cases, such as if you have a heart pacemaker or are in the early stages of pregnancy.

If you wish to try TENS, and your doctor agrees that it is suitable for you, you might be able to try a machine for free. If you find it effective, you will need to purchase your own, but make sure you buy one from a reputable source and get proper instructions on how to use it.

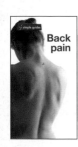

Back pain

For more information see
Back pain

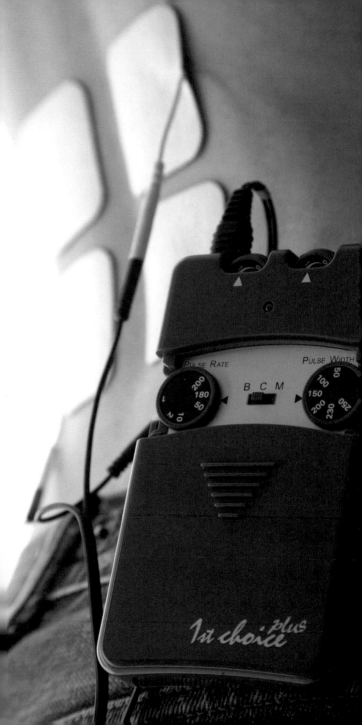

Massage

Gentle massage can have many benefits for people with arthritis. By warming the affected area, massage can help to relax muscles, reduce inflammation and ease pain. Of course you can massage your own muscles, but many people prefer to undergo regular massage sessions with a qualified professional. Always make sure that you tell your therapist about your arthritis before embarking on any course of treatment.

Heat and cold treatments

Many people find that applying heat or cold to the affected area helps to relieve the pain of arthritis. Whilst heat helps to relax the muscles, coldness can numb the affected area and reduce swelling. You may find that your symptoms respond well to:

- heating pads and lamps

- a warm bath or a jacuzzi

- an electric blanket or a hot water bottle

- an ice pack (make your own by wrapping a towel round a bag of frozen peas).

Dietary supplements

Supplements like glucosamine and chondroitin may have a role to play in relieving the pain associated with osteoarthritis. Some people choose to take the two supplements together. The effectiveness of these substances (which are available as tablets from most health food shops or pharmacies) is currently being investigated in clinical trials conducted in large groups of people with arthritis. We will know more when the results of these trials become available.

Always keep your doctor informed of any supplements you are using to control your arthritis, in case these interfere with the programme of care that they are recommending.

SPECIAL TREATMENT GROUPS

Arthritis in children

Arthritis can affect people of any age, and children are no exception. About one in every 1,000 children has arthritis, and this often takes the form of juvenile idiopathic arthritis (JIA). **Juvenile** means that the arthritis began before the age of 16 and **idiopathic** means that the cause is not known. There are three common types of juvenile idiopathic arthritis:

- **Pauciarticular arthritis**
  Affects a maximum of four joints, which become swollen and painful. The eyes can also be affected.

- **Polyarthritis**
  Affects five or more joints. Usually spreads from one joint to another fairly rapidly.

- **Systemic disease**
  Affects the whole body and causes fever and rashes as well as inflamed and painful joints.

Arthritis is diagnosed in children in much the same way as it is in adults, by performing a physical examination, looking at the child's range of movement and by carrying out certain tests, likes blood analyses and scans. Juvenile arthritis is treated with the same medications and therapies that are used in adults.

- NSAIDs and corticosteroid injections to reduce inflammation of the joints.

- DMARDs to try to slow down the progression of the disease.

- Regular exercise to build muscle strength and control weight.

- Physiotherapy to keep joints flexible and to maintain muscle strength.

Given the right treatment, children with arthritis can expect to lead normal lives, both during their childhood and as they move into adulthood. Many children affected by juvenile arthritis find that their symptoms disappear altogether as they get older.

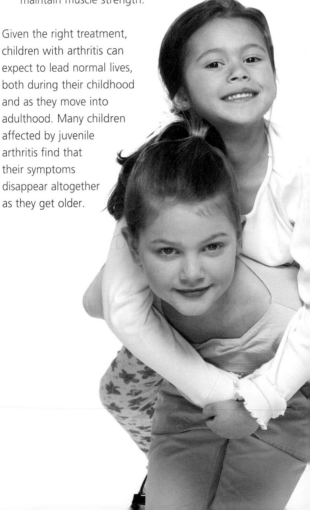

ARTHRITIS AND PREGNANCY

Many women with rheumatoid arthritis find that their symptoms disappear whilst they are pregnant (only to return after they have given birth). No-one is quite sure why this is.

Of course, it stands to reason that as your pregnancy progresses and your weight gradually increases, the amount of pressure that your joints are under will also increase quite significantly.

The hormones you produce whilst you are pregnant can also affect your joints. Some pregnancy hormones cause the ligaments between the pelvic bones to soften and your joints to loosen in preparation for the birth. As the structures that support your pelvic organs become more flexible, you may feel considerable discomfort on either side of your lower back.

There are a number of steps that women can take to avoid joint pain whilst they are pregnant:

- wear low-heeled shoes with good arch support

- sleep on your side with a pillow between your legs

- use a support belt to take some of the weight of your baby away from your back

- do pelvic tilts (involves contracting your tummy muscles whilst tucking your bottom down and under your spine) to strengthen the pelvis and reduce lower back pain

- take warm baths or use a warm jet of water from a shower head on the affected area

- exercise regularly (but always consult your doctor before starting any exercise routine).

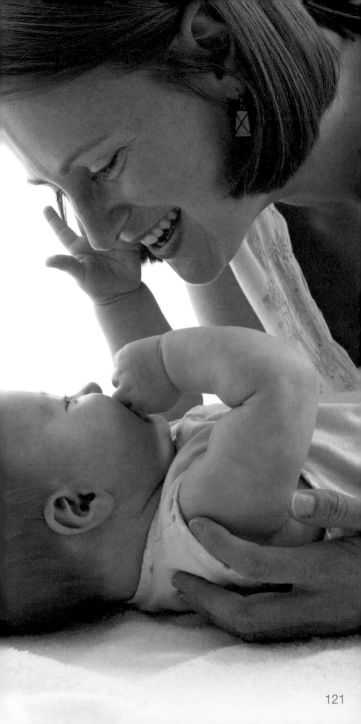

THE LONG AND SHORT OF IT

At its worst, arthritis can leave you in a lot of pain and by preventing you from getting around and carrying out certain activities, can start to make you feel very dependent on other people. However, this needn't always be the case. Although arthritis cannot be cured, there are many things you can do, and medications you can take, to help ease the pain and discomfort of arthritis and preserve your functioning (and therefore your independence).

One of the most important things you can do is to try and remain positive, and make sure that you feel in control of your arthritis, not the other way around. Keep talking to people about your arthritis, whether it is your family, your friends, your colleagues, your doctor or fellow sufferers.

Whether you are managed by your GP at your local surgery or referred to an arthritis specialist, be assured that you are in the best possible hands. Listen to what they tell you, take it seriously and try to adhere to the programme of care that they recommend. Although a complete cure may be difficult to achieve, you should be able to live with your arthritis without it restricting your lifestyle significantly. Most importantly, you should not allow pain to control the way in which you live your life.

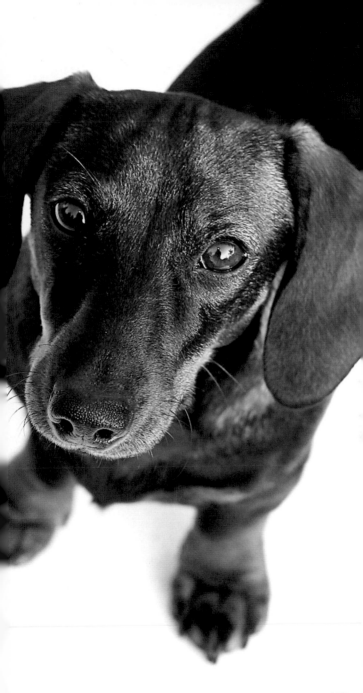

GETTING THE MOST OUT OF YOUR HEALTH SERVICE

Arthritis is a long-term condition and it is important that you work together with your doctor to optimise your care. Maintaining a good relationship with your GP, specialist or any other healthcare member you may come into contact with, is fundamental to managing your arthritis effectively. These people will be able to explain to you why you are in pain, teach you how best to manage your pain and help to relieve your pain by physical manipulation, drug treatment, or in the most severe cases, surgery. It is important that you remain in regular contact with your GP, and keep them informed of any improvement or deterioration in your symptoms. Remember, if one management approach fails to work, there are many others that can be tried.

- Don't be afraid to ask for help or advice.

- Keep your doctor informed of all the treatments you are taking, including dietary supplements.

- Know what to expect and when to ask for help.

- Consider bringing a carer along to your doctor's appointments so that they can be kept up to speed on any changes to your care programme.

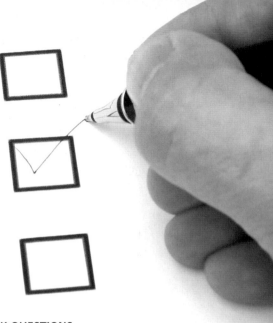

ASK QUESTIONS

Having a doctor's appointment or going to the hospital for tests can be quite a daunting prospect. It is often helpful to write down a list of questions before you attend your appointment.

- What type of arthritis do I have?

- How severe is my arthritis?

- It is likely to get worse?

- Do I need to have any tests?

- What type of treatment suits me best?

- What should I do if the treatment doesn't make me feel better?

- Can I carry on going to work?

- Are there any exercises that can help?

- Are there any alternative or complementary therapies that might help?

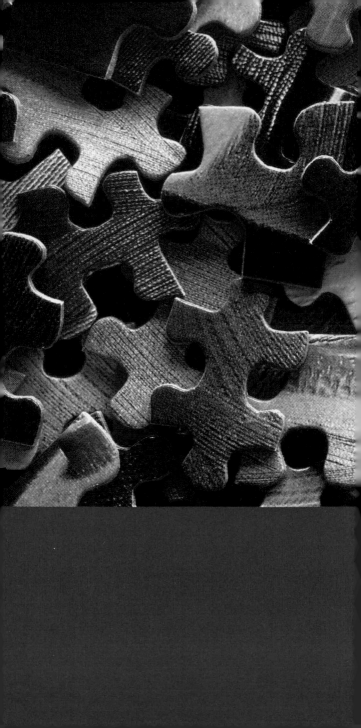

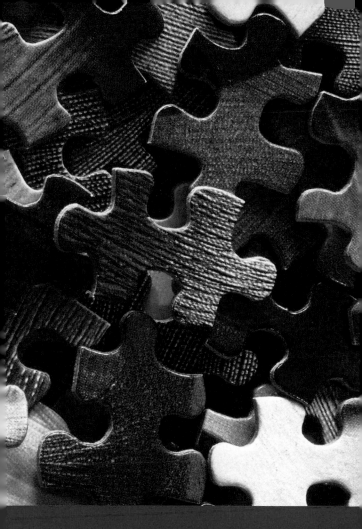

**Simple
extras**

FURTHER READING

■ *Back Pain (Simple Guide)*
CSF Medical Communications Ltd, 2005
ISBN: 1-905466-01-3, £5.99
www.bestmedicine.com

■ *Cholesterol (Simple Guide)*
CSF Medical Communications Ltd, 2005
ISBN: 1-905466-05-6, £5.99
www.bestmedicine.com

■ *Osteoporosis (Simple Guide)*
CSF Medical Communications Ltd, 2006
ISBN: 1-905466-11-0, £5.99
www.bestmedicine.com

■ *Thyroid disorders (Simple Guide)*
CSF Medical Communications Ltd, 2006
ISBN: 1-905466-09-9, £5.99
www.bestmedicine.com

USEFUL CONTACTS

■ Age Concern England
Astral House
1268 London Road
London
SW16 4ER
Helpline: 0800 009966
Website: *www.ace.org.uk*

■ **The Arthritic Association**
One Upperton Gardens
Eastbourne
East Sussex
BN21 2AA
Tel: 0800 652 3188
Website: *www.arthriticassociation.org.uk*

■ **Arthritis Care**
18 Stephenson Way
London
NW1 2HD
Helpline: 0808 8000 4050
Tel: 020 7380 6500
Website: *www.arthritiscare.org.uk*

■ **Arthritis Research Campaign (ARC)**
Copeman House
St Mary's Court
St Mary's Gate
Chesterfield
Derbyshire
S41 7TD
Tel: 0870 850 5000
Website: *www.arc.org.uk*

■ **Benefits Enquiry Line (BEL)**
Tel: 0800 882200
Website: *www.dwp.gov.uk*

- **British Acupuncture Council (BAcC)**
  63 Jeddo Road
  London
  W12 9HQ
  Tel: 020 8735 0400
  Website: *www.acupuncture.org.uk*

- **British Orthopaedic Association**
  35–43 Lincoln's Inn Fields
  London
  WC2A 3PN
  Tel: 020 7405 6507
  Website: *www.boa.ac.uk*

- **The British Pain Society**
  21 Portland Place
  London
  W1B 1PY
  Tel: 020 7631 8870
  Website: *www.britishpainsociety.org*

- **British Society for Rheumatology**
  Bride House
  18–20 Bride Lane
  London
  EC4Y 8EE
  Tel: 020 7842 0900
  Website: *www.rheumatology.org.uk*

- **Carers UK**
  Ruth Pitter House
  20/25 Glasshouse Yard
  London
  EC1A 4JP
  Tel: 0808 808 7777
  Website: *www.carersuk.org*

- **Chartered Society of Physiotherapy**
  14 Bedford Row
  London
  WC1R 4ED
  Tel: 020 7306 6666
  Website: *www.csp.org.uk*

- **Citizens Advice Bureau (CAB)**
  Website: *www.citizensadvice.org.uk*

- **College of Occupational Therapists**
  106–114 Borough High Street
  Southwark
  London
  SE1 1LB
  Tel: 020 7357 6480
  Website: *www.cot.org.uk*

- **Counsel and Care**
  Twyman House
  16 Bonny Street
  London
  NW1 9PG
  Advice line: 0845 300 7585
  Website: *www.counselandcare.org.uk*

- **Dial UK (Disability Information & Advice Line)**
  St Catherine's
  Tickhill Road
  Doncaster
  South Yorks
  Tel: 01302 310123
  Website: *www.dialuk.org.uk*

■ **Disability Alliance**
Universal House
88–94 Wentworth Street
London
E1 7SA
Tel: 020 7247 8776
Website: *www.disabilityalliance.org*

■ **Disabled Living Foundation (DLF)**
380–384 Harrow Road
London
W9 2HU
Tel: 0845 130 9177
Website: *www.dlf.org.uk*

■ **Disability Rights Commission (DRC)**
FREEPOST
MID02164
Stratford upon Avon
CV37 9BR
Tel: 08457 622633
Website: *www.drc-gb.org*

■ **Motability**
Motability Operations
City Gate House
22 Southwark Bridge Road
London
SE1 9HB
Tel: 0845 456 4566
Website: *www.motability.co.uk*

■ **NHS Direct**
NHS Direct Line: 0845 46 47
Website: *www.nhsdirect.nhs.uk*

■ **Motability Advice and Vehicle Information Service (MAVIS)**
Crowthorne Business Estate
Old Wokingham Road
Crowthorne
Berks
RG45 6XD
Tel: 01344 661000
Website: *www.dft.gov.uk/access/mavis*

■ **National Rheumatoid Arthritis Society (NRAS)**
Unit B4 Westacott Business Centre
Westacott Way
Littlewick Green
Maidenhead
SL6 3RT
Tel: 0845 458 3969
Website: *www.rheumatoid.org.uk*

YOUR RIGHTS

As a patient, you have a number of important rights. These include the right to the best possible standard of care, the right to information, the right to dignity and respect, the right to confidentiality and underpinning all of these, the right to good health.

Occasionally, you may feel as though your rights have been compromised, or you may be unsure of where you stand when it comes to qualifying for certain treatments or services. In these instances, there are a number of organisations you can turn to for help and advice. Remember that lodging a complaint against your health service should not compromise the quality of care you receive, either now or in the future.

■ **The Patients Association**
The Patients Association (*www.patients-association.com*) is a UK charity which represents patient rights, influences health policy and campaigns for better patient care.
Contact details:
PO Box 935
Harrow
Middlesex
HA1 3YJ
Helpline: 0845 6084455
Email: *mailbox@patients-association.com*

■ **Citizens Advice Bureau**
The Citizens Advice Bureau (*www.nacab.org.uk*) provides free, independent and confidential advice to NHS patients at a number of outreach centres located throughout the country (*www.adviceguide.org.uk*).
Contact details:
Find your local Citizens Advice Bureau using the search tool at *www.citizensadvice.org.uk*.

■ **Patient Advice and Liaison Services (PALS)**

Set up by the Department of Health (*www.dh.gov.uk*), PALS provide information, support and confidential advice to patients, families and their carers.

Contact details:

Phone your local hospital, clinic, GP surgery or health centre and ask for details of the PALS, or call NHS Direct on 0845 46 47.

■ **The Independent Complaints Advocacy Service (ICAS)**

ICAS is an independent service that can help you bring about formal complaints against your NHS practitioner. ICAS provides support, help, advice and advocacy from experienced advisors and caseworkers.

Contact details:

ICAS Central Team
Myddelton House
115–123 Pentonville Road
London N1 9LZ
Email: *icascentralteam@citizensadvice.org.uk*
Or contact your local ICAS office direct.

Accessing your medical records

You have a legal right to see all your health records under the Data Protection Act of 1998. You can usually make an informal request to your doctor and you should be given access within 40 days. Note that you may have to pay a small fee for the privilege.

You can be denied access to your records if your doctor believes that the information contained within them could cause serious harm to you or another person. If you are applying for access on behalf of someone else, then you will not be granted access to information which the patient gave to his or her doctor on the understanding that it would remain confidential remain confidential.

Regional Public Services Ombudsmen
The Health Service Ombudsman for England
Millbank Tower
Millbank
London
SW1P 4QP
Tel: 0845 015 4033 (Minicom 020 7217 4066)
Email: *phso.enquiries@ombudsman.org.uk*
Website: *www.ombudsman.org.uk*

The Public Services Ombudsman for Wales
1 Ffordd yr Hen Gae
Pencoed
CF35 5LJ
Tel: 01656 641 150
Email: *ask@ombudsman-wales.org.uk*
Website: *www.ombudsman-wales.org*

The Scottish Public Services Ombudsman
4 Melville Street
Edinburgh
EH3 7NS
Tel: 0870 011 5378 (Text: 0790 049 4372)
Email: *enquiries@scottishombudsman.org.uk*
Website: *www.scottishombudsman.org.uk/contact*

Northern Ireland Ombudsman
Freepost
BEL 1478
Belfast BT1 6BR
Tel: 0800 343424 (free) or 028 9023 3821
Email: *ombudsman@ni-ombudsman.org.uk*
Website: *www.ni-ombudsman.org.uk*

SIMPLE GUIDE QUESTIONNAIRE

Dear reader,

We would love to know what you thought of this Simple Guide. Please take a few moments to fill out this short questionnaire and return it to us at the FREEPOST address below.

CSF Medical Communications Ltd
FREEPOST NAT5703
Witney
OX29 8BR

SO WHAT DID YOU THINK?

Which Simple Guide have you just read?

_____

Where did you buy it (store/town)?

_____

Who did you buy it for?

☐ Myself ☐ Friend ☐ Relative
☐ Patient ☐ Other

Where did you hear about the Simple Guides?

☐ They were recommended to me ☐ Internet
☐ Stumbled across them ☐ Other

Did it meet with your expectations?

☐ Exceeded ☐ Met all
☐ Met most ☐ Fell below

Was there anything you particularly liked?

_____

_____

_____

Was there anything we could have improved?

_____

_____

_____

WHO ARE YOU?

Name: _____

Address: _____

_____

_____

Tel: _____

Email: _____

How old are you?
☐ Under 25   ☐ 25–34   ☐ 35–44
☐ 45–54   ☐ 55–64   ☐ 65+

Are you...   ☐ Male   ☐ Female

Do you suffer from a long-term medical condition? If so, please specify.

_____

WHAT NEXT?

What other topics would you like to see covered in future Simple Guides?

Thanks,
the Simple Guides team